# Controversies in Thoracic Surgery

*Editors*

LANA Y. SCHUMACHER
DAVID C. GRIFFIN

# THORACIC SURGERY CLINICS

www.thoracic.theclinics.com

*Consulting Editor*
VIRGINIA R. LITLE

May 2023 • Volume 33 • Number 2

**ELSEVIER**

1600 John F. Kennedy Boulevard • Suite 1800 • Philadelphia, Pennsylvania, 19103-2899

http://www.thoracic.theclinics.com

**THORACIC SURGERY CLINICS Volume 33, Number 2**
**May 2023 ISSN 1547-4127, ISBN-13: 978-0-323-93931-7**

**Editor:** John Vassallo (j.vassallo@elsevier.com)
**Developmental Editor:** Jessica Nicole B. Cañaberal

*Thoracic Surgery Clinics* (ISSN 1547-4127) is published quarterly by Elsevier Inc., 360 Park Avenue South, New York, NY 10010-1710. Months of publication are February, May, August, and November. Business and editorial offices: 1600 John F. Kennedy Boulevard, Suite 1800, Philadelphia, PA 19103-2899. Periodicals postage paid at New York, NY, and additional mailing offices. Subscription prices are $417.00 per year (US individuals), $681.00 per year (US institutions), $100.00 per year (US students), $487.00 per year (Canadian individuals), $881.00 per year (Canadian institutions), $100.00 per year (Canadian students), $225.00 per year (international students), $509.00 per year (international individuals), and $881.00 per year (international institutions). Foreign air speed delivery is included in all Clinics' subscription prices. All prices are subject to change without notice. **POSTMASTER:** Send address changes to Thoracic Surgery Clinics, Elsevier Health Sciences Division, Subscription Customer Service, 3251 Riverport Lane, Maryland Heights, MO 63043. **Customer Service (orders, claims, online, change of address): Telephone: 1-800-654-2452 (U.S. and Canada); 314-447-8871 (outside U.S. and Canada). Fax: 314-447-8029. E-mail: journalscustomerservice-usa@elsevier.com (for print support); journalsonlinesupport-usa@elsevier.com (for online support).**

*Reprints.* For copies of 100 or more, of articles in this publication, please contact Commercial Rights Department, Elsevier Inc., 360 Park Avenue South, New York, NY 10010-1710. Tel: 212-633-3874; Fax: 212-633-3820; E-mail: reprints@elsevier.com.

*Thoracic Surgery Clinics* is covered in *MEDLINE/PubMed (Index Medicus), EMBASE/Excerpta Medica, Science Citation Index Expanded (SciSearch®), Journal Citation Reports/Science Edition,* and *Current Contents®/Clinical Medicine.*

# Contributors

## CONSULTING EDITOR

**VIRGINIA R. LITLE, MD**
Chief of Thoracic Surgery, SMG Thoracic
Surgery, Brighton, Massachusetts, USA

## EDITORS

**LANA SCHUMACHER, MD, MS, FACS**
Director of Robotic Thoracic Surgery, Program
Director of Robotic Surgical Education,
Division of Thoracic Surgery, Department of
Surgery, Massachusetts General Hospital,
Boston, Massachusetts, USA

**DAVID GRIFFIN, MD, FACS**
Thoracic Surgeon, Intermountain Health,
Murray, Utah, USA

## AUTHORS

**MARA B. ANTONOFF, MD, FACS**
Department of Thoracic and Cardiovascular
Surgery, The University of Texas MD Anderson
Cancer Center, Houston, Texas, USA

**CARLY C. BARRON, MD, MSc**
Medical Oncology Training Program, University
of Toronto, Division of Medical Oncology,
Princess Margaret Cancer Centre, Toronto,
Ontario, Canada

**DARREN S. BRYAN, MD**
Assistant Professor Surgery, Section of
Thoracic Surgery, Department of Surgery,
University of Chicago Medicine, Chicago,
Illinois, USA

**MICAELA LANGILLE COLLINS, MD, MPH**
General Surgery Resident, Department of
Surgery, Thomas Jefferson University Hospital,
Philadelphia, Pennsylvania, USA

**NATHANIEL DEBOEVER, MD**
Department of Thoracic and Cardiovascular
Surgery, The University of Texas MD Anderson
Cancer Center, Houston, Texas, USA

**JESSICA S. DONINGTON, MD**
Professor of Surgery, Chief, Section of
Thoracic Surgery, Department of Surgery,
University of Chicago Medicine, Chicago,
Illinois, USA

**MICHAEL EISENBERG, MD**
Department of Thoracic and Cardiovascular
Surgery, The University of Texas MD Anderson
Cancer Center, Houston, Texas, USA

**ELENA ELIMOVA, MD, MSc**
Division of Medical Oncology, Princess
Margaret Cancer Centre, Toronto, Ontario,
Canada

**KELLY FAIRBAIRN, DO**
Clinical Fellow, Division of Cardiothoracic
Surgery, University of Arizona, Tucson,
Arizona, USA

**HIRAN C. FERNANDO, MBBS, FRCS**
Department of Cardiothoracic Surgery,
Allegheny General Hospital, Pittsburgh,
Pennsylvania, USA

**FRANK GLEASON, MD, MSPH**
Department of Surgery, The University of Alabama at Birmingham, Birmingham, Alabama, USA

**MATTHEW L. INRA, MD**
Lenox Hill Hospital at Northwell Health, New York, New York, USA

**MIN P. KIM, MD**
Vice-Chair of Department of Surgery, David M. Underwood Distinguished Professor of Surgery, Professor of Surgery and Cardiothoracic Surgery at Weill Cornell Medicine, Houston Methodist Hospital, Houston, Texas, USA

**RICHARD LAZZARO, MD**
Chief, Thoracic Surgery, Southern Region Robert Wood Johnson Barnabas Health, New Brunswick, New Jersey, USA

**CONOR M. MAXWELL, DO**
Department of Surgery, Allegheny General Hospital, Pittsburgh, Pennsylvania, USA

**CALVIN NG, MBBS (Hons), MD (Res) (Lond), FRCSEd, FCSHK, FHKAM (Surg), FCCP, FAPSR**
Department of Surgery, Prince of Wales Hospital, Shatin, New Territories, Hong Kong

**OLUGBENGA OKUSANYA, MD, FACS**
Assistant Professor, Division of Thoracic Surgery, Department of Surgery, Thomas Jefferson University Hospital, Philadelphia, Pennsylvania, USA

**NIKHIL PANDA, MD, MPH**
Division of Thoracic Surgery, Department of Surgery, Massachusetts General Hospital, Boston, Massachusetts, USA

**SIVA RAJA, MD, PhD**
Staff Surgeon, Thoracic Surgery, Thoracic and Cardiovascular Surgery Institute, Cleveland Clinic Foundation, Cleveland, Ohio, USA

**LANA SCHUMACHER, MD, MS, FACS**
Director of Robotic Thoracic Surgery, Program Director of Robotic Surgical Education, Division of Thoracic Surgery, Department of Surgery, Massachusetts General Hospital, Boston, Massachusetts, USA

**ANUJ SHAH, MD**
General Surgery Resident, Houston Methodist Hospital, Houston, Texas, USA

**MONISHA SUDARSHAN, MD, MPH**
Staff Surgeon, Thoracic Surgery, Thoracic and Cardiovascular Surgery Institute, Cleveland Clinic Foundation, Cleveland, Ohio, USA

**SADIA TASNIM, MD**
Digestive Disease and Surgery Institute, Thoracic and Cardiovascular Surgery Institute, Cleveland Clinic Foundation, Cleveland, Ohio, USA

**XIN WANG, MD, PhD**
Medical Oncology Training Program, University of Toronto, Division of Medical Oncology, Princess Margaret Cancer Centre, Toronto, Ontario, Canada

**BENJAMIN WEI, MD**
Associate Professor, Department of Surgery, Division of Cardiothoracic Surgery, The University of Alabama at Birmingham, Birmingham Veterans Administration Medical Center, Birmingham, Alabama, USA

**STEPHANIE G. WORRELL, MD**
Thoracic Section Chief, Clinical Assistant Professor, Department of Surgery, University of Arizona, Tucson, Arizona, USA

# Contents

Esophageal perforation is a rare but fatal disease process that requires prompt diagnosis and treatment. Surgery has historically been required for treatment; however, there is currently a shift toward endoscopic management. Although no randomized controlled trials exist to compare patient outcomes, many case series and systematic analyses describe their indications, efficacy, and safety profile. Endoscopic stenting and endoscopic vacuum therapy are the 2 therapies most widely described across a diverse patient population and appear to be safe and effective when treating esophageal perforation, in the proper clinical setting. Guidelines and scoring systems exist to help direct management and stratify patient risk.

Gastroesophageal reflux disease (GERD) is among the most prevalent diseases in the United States. Despite mainstay therapy of lifestyle modifications and medical therapy, GERD necessitates testing to determine if invasive therapy will improve symptoms. Gold standard therapy is minimally invasive fundoplication. Patients with body mass index <35, small or no hiatal hernia, normal motility, and pathologic GERD should consider magnetic sphincter augmentation. Endoscopic treatment with either Stretta or Transoral Incisionless fundoplication 2.0 must be considered if surgery is undesirable. Outcomes of endoscopic treatments are better compared with medical therapy but worse than surgical therapy.

Approaches to achalasia include non-operative and operative techniques with Heller Myotomy and Per-Oral Endoscopic Myotomy (POEM) at the forefront of palliative strategies. Given the diverse subtypes and the time-dependent failure pattern for achalasia, there is no standard approach. We elect for a POEM for type III achalasia, poor functional status, hostile abdomen, and salvage after the previous myotomy. A Heller myotomy is elected over a POEM for type II achalasia, presence of diverticulum, and hiatal hernia. As long-term outcomes become available, an optimal customized strategy will become clearer.

Video content accompanies this article at http://www.thoracic.theclinics.com.

Tracheobronchomalacia (TBM) is an increasingly recognized abnormality of the central airways in patients with respiratory symptoms. Severe TBM in symptomatic patients warrants screening dynamic CT of the chest and/or awake dynamic bronchoscopy. The goal of surgical repair is to restore the C-shaped configuration of the airway lumen and splint or secure the lax posterior membrane to the mesh to ameliorate symptoms. Robotic tracheobronchoplasty is safe and associated with improvements in pulmonary function and subjective improvement in quality of life.

The lung represents the most common site for metastatic spread of extrathoracic primary malignancies. Pulmonary metastatic disease occurs in a wide breadth of cancers with a multitude of histologies, and, historically, has been managed predominantly with systemic therapy. However, in appropriately selected patients, pulmonary metastasectomy can provide extended disease-free intervals, relief from systemic therapy, and prolonged survival. Thus, pulmonary metastasectomy serves a vital role in the armamentarium against a multitude of primary malignancies. Moreover, as systemic agents improve and more patients live longer with stage IV cancer, pulmonary metastasectomy will likely have increasing relevance in the future.

Bronchopulmonary carcinoid tumors are rare, well-differentiated neuroendocrine neoplasms. They can be categorized as typical or atypical lesions and are low-to-intermediate-grade, respectively. The cornerstone of therapy for carcinoid tumors is surgical resection and current consensus guidelines recommend anatomic resection for stage I to IIIA disease. The renewed interest in sublobar resections for the treatment of lung malignancies has sparked debate over the degree of resection necessary for these indolent lesions. Segmentectomy provides an oncologic resection while preserving as much lung parenchyma as possible, and is a reasonable approach to apply to small, undifferentiated, or typical carcinoid lesions.

Sublobar resections are commonly performed operations that have seen an increase in applicability. The sublobar approach, comprising segmentectomy and wedge resections, can provide lung preservation and thus is better tolerated in select patients in comparison to lobectomy. These operations are offered for a variety of benign and malignant lesions. Understanding the indications and technical aspects of these approaches is paramount as improvements in lung cancer screening protocols and the imaging modalities has led to an increase in the detection of early-stage cancer. In this article, we discuss the anatomy, indications, technical approaches, and outcomes for sublobar resection.

# THORACIC SURGERY CLINICS

---

### SERIES OF RELATED INTEREST

*Advances in Surgery*
http://www.advancessurgery.com/

*Surgical Clinics*
http://www.surgical.theclinics.com/

*Surgical Oncology Clinics*
https://www.surgonc.theclinics.com/

---

**THE CLINICS ARE AVAILABLE ONLINE!**
Access your subscription at:
www.theclinics.com

# Foreword
# Thoracic Surgery: Where's the Controversy?

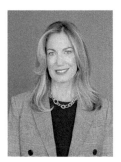

Virginia R. Litle, MD
*Consulting Editor*

What's controversial in our field? Aren't we all on the same page when it comes to patient care? No, we're not; thus, Drs Lana Schumacher and David Griffin have offered up 12 areas where management may differ between thoracic surgeons or between surgeons and their medical specialty colleagues. The evidence doesn't always support one consensus, and (apparently) there can be more than one way to skin a cat, so they say. With relevance to us, however, in the operating room and clinic is that there may be several ways to approach esophageal, lung, airway, and mediastinal disease, but robust evidence lends guidance for best clinical practice.

In this issue of *Thoracic Surgery Clinics*, invited experts provide current data to help you navigate sometimes muddy waters. Drs Lazzaro and Inra share with us the value of working up patients with chronic cough, chronic obstructive pulmonary disease, and suspected tracheobronchomalacia. Collaborating with interventional and general pulmonologists to identify patients who may benefit from a workup and subsequent intervention, specifically robotic tracheobronchoplasty, can improve quality of life for these patients.

Oncologic management can be particularly challenging in the era of relatively speedy advances in systemic therapy for both lung and esophageal cancer and at a time when patients carry around an encyclopedia of knowledge in their back pocket. Dr Donington is one of our thoracic experts in the area of targeted and immunotherapy for lung cancer, so we welcome her thoughts with coauthor Dr Bryan, as they summarize how to approach stage IIIA non–small cell lung cancer. Unfortunately, the activity in this space contributes to even more controversies as they summarize: "…resectability, use of pneumonectomy, value of adjuvant versus neoadjuvant therapy and need to reassess the mediastinum prior to resection." No shortage of research topics there! With regards to the early high-risk lung cancer patients, Dr Fernando has been addressing tumor ablation for years, and so he shares his thoughts with coauthors Drs Maxwell and Ng. Essentially, we look forward to the results of stereotactic radiation therapy versus resection randomized trials, and we should appreciate, and be involved in, the continued progress in bronchoscopic ablative therapies. Remember that advanced bronchoscopic training for surgeons is out there, although working with interventional pulmonology may be an efficient practice option as well.

Dr Antonoff has committed much research and mentoring time to investigating the area of pulmonary metastasectomy. Drs Eisenberg, Deboever and Dr Antonoff remind us that even in the era of immunotherapy, there is a role for metastasectomy, and for the time being the principle of controlling the primary and resecting all the metastases still should be used.

In the arena of benign esophagus, there's never a shortage of discussion topics, including peroral endoscopic myotomy versus surgical myotomy for achalasia and how to manage gastroesophageal reflux disease (GERD). The value of a regularly scheduled benign esophagus conference,

Thorac Surg Clin 33 (2023) ix–x
https://doi.org/10.1016/j.thorsurg.2023.02.001
1547-4127/23/© 2023 Published by Elsevier Inc.

including the interventional, neurogastroenterologists, and community gastroenterologists, cannot be undervalued for thoracic surgeons with benign foregut practices. Dr Raja and colleagues at Cleveland Clinic share their expert insight on achalasia management, reflecting the busy practice there established by Dr Tom Rice and colleagues. And in this *Thoracic Surgery Clinics* issue, Dr Kim summarizes endoscopic approaches for GERD, an ever-evolving area in which techniques seem to pass distally as long-term results are reported.

Understanding the controversies and having data both aid in the shared decision-making conversations with patients, the discussion at multidisciplinary tumor boards as well as in resident education. Thank you to the excellent work and time of *all* the contributing authors and to the guest editors Drs Schumacher and Griffin. We hope this issue clears the water and helps you optimize patient care and satisfaction. Enjoy!

Sincerely,

Virginia R. Litle, MD
SMG Thoracic Surgery
736 Cambridge Street
Brighton, MA 02135, USA

*E-mail address:*
vlitle@gmail.com

Twitter: @vlitlemd (V.R. Litle)

# Preface
# The More Things Change...

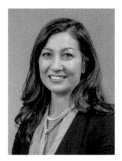
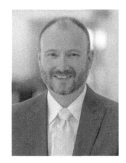

Lana Schumacher, MD, MS, FACS    David Griffin, MD, FACS
*Editors*

It is our great pleasure to introduce the latest issue of *Thoracic Surgery Clinics* entitled "Controversies in Thoracic Surgery." Surgical technique continues to evolve, and increased adoption of minimally invasive techniques drive improvements in surgical care. Furthermore, exciting advances in collaborative fields, such as medical oncology and gastrointestinal endoscopy, have dramatically impacted how we practice as thoracic surgeons and have, in some cases, kept us (and our patients) out of the operating room.

Although much has changed in our field since the last Controversies issue was published in 2016, many of the same vexing questions remain. The nature of surgical care makes it difficult to generate level one evidence, the holy grail of medical decision making, and mandates us to rely on systematic retrospective reviews and expert opinion in many cases to make decisions. As you know, this level of evidence innately generates controversy about the best treatment path for our patients given the inherent limitations.[1]

The following well-written articles from content experts touch on the full breadth and depth of thoracic surgery and detail exactly how these changes impact our decision making. We are hopeful that you will find these articles useful for answering the difficult but exceedingly common questions in general thoracic surgery.

These questions include how best to incorporate novel immunotherapy agents in the treatment of common thoracic malignancies, best practices for metastasectomy as well as endoscopic advances in the treatment of benign esophageal disease, such as reflux and achalasia. Furthermore, other authors describe the current understanding of the long-standing controversy in thoracic surgery, pulmonary resection versus radiotherapy for early-stage lung cancer in high-risk patients.

We would like to thank all of the authors and contributors for their well-researched and insightful articles. We would also like to thank Dr Litle and the publishing team at Elsevier for their invaluable assistance, mentorship, and support.

Lana Schumacher, MD, MS, FACS
Massachusetts General Hospital
55 Fruit Street, Austen 7
Boston, MA 02114, USA

David Griffin, MD, FACS
Intermountain Health
5169 South Cottonwood Street
Murray, UT 84107, USA

*E-mail addresses:*
lschumacher2@mgh.harvard.edu
(L. Schumacher)
David.Griffin@imail.org (D. Griffin)

## REFERENCE

1. Knight SR. The value of systemic meta-analyses in surgery. Eur Surg Res 2021;62:221–8.

Thorac Surg Clin 33 (2023) xi
https://doi.org/10.1016/j.thorsurg.2023.02.002
1547-4127/23/© 2023 Published by Elsevier Inc.

# Esophageal Perforation
## Is Surgery Still Necessary?

Kelly Fairbairn, DO, Stephanie G. Worrell, MD*

## KEYWORDS

- Esophageal perforation • Esophageal stent • Endoscopic vacuum therapy • Esophageal surgery

## KEY POINTS

- Esophageal perforation is a rare but serious disease process that can lead to mediastinitis and death.
- Treatment of esophageal perforation is moving toward conservative, endoscopic techniques such as stenting and endoscopic vacuum therapy.
- No randomized controlled trials exist comparing surgery with endoscopic therapies.
- Self-expanding metal stents and endoscopic vacuum therapy seem to be safe and effective treatment strategies for esophageal perforation in the proper clinical setting.

## INTRODUCTION

Esophageal perforation is relatively uncommon, with an incidence of 3.1/1000000 a year,[1] and is potentially fatal if not promptly diagnosed and properly treated. Mortality from esophageal perforation doubles after a 24-hour delay in diagnosis,[2] with the natural history of the disease leading to necrotizing mediastinitis and/or sepsis. The causes of perforation vary. Historically, prompt surgical intervention was the treatment of choice for all esophageal perforations; however, new endoscopic therapies have evolved that are challenging that dictum. To date, no randomized controlled trials exist to guide management. A discussion of esophageal perforation and the optimum treatment strategy follows.

## PHYSIOLOGY

The esophagus has 3 anatomical points of narrowing—the cricopharyngeus muscle, the bronchoaortic constriction, and the gastroesophageal junction—and has a predilection for perforation at these sites. A lack of a serosal layer and increased intraluminal pressure, especially at these anatomic sites of narrowing, or narrowing from malignancy, foreign body, or physiologic dysfunction can all lead to rupture. Rupture leads to leakage of the esophagogastric contents into the mediastinum, which creates a necrotizing inflammatory process leading to sepsis, multiorgan failure, and death without proper intervention.[3,4]

The cause of esophageal perforation varies, making a proper clinical history imperative. More than half of perforations in adults are iatrogenic, most commonly from complex upper endoscopy (**Fig. 1**). Following iatrogenic cause is Boerhaave syndrome (15% of presentation), foreign body obstruction (12%), trauma (9%), intraoperative injury (2%), and malignancy (1%). Other less common causes include caustic ingestion, pneumatic injury, peptic ulceration, Crohn disease, and eosinophilic esophagitis.[2]

### Clinical Presentation and Evaluation

The clinical presentation of esophageal perforation will vary based on the cause and location of the perforation, as well as the length of time since the perforation. Cervical perforation can present with neck pain, erythema, and edema, whereas thoracic perforations can present with chest pain, and gastroesophageal junction perforations

Department of Surgery, Section of Thoracic Surgery, University of Arizona, 1501 North Campbell Avenue, Tucson, AZ 85724, USA
* Corresponding author.
*E-mail address:* SWorrell@Arizona.edu

Thorac Surg Clin 33 (2023) 117–123
https://doi.org/10.1016/j.thorsurg.2023.01.005
1547-4127/23/© 2023 Elsevier Inc. All rights reserved.

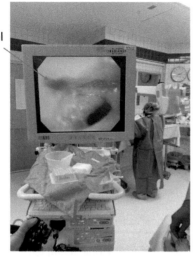

Esophageal lumen

**Fig. 1.** Cervical perforation at the time of endoscopic retrograde cholangiopancreatography. Esophageal lumen (*blue arrow*).

can present with either chest or abdominal pain or both. All patients can present with subcutaneous emphysema and signs of sepsis and multiorgan failure.

A thorough history and physical examination should be the first step in the patient workup. In any patient presenting with mediastinal air, a high index of suspicion should be maintained, as the consequences of missing an esophageal injury are severe and carry a poor prognosis. Questions regarding food ingestion, vomiting, esophageal instrumentation, and trauma, as well as a full medical history should be obtained. A full set of laboratory results including a complete blood count, basic metabolic panel, and a type and screen should be drawn. Electrolyte abnormalities may be seen with a history of severe vomiting. Imaging will be directed based on the suspected location of perforation and often includes a computed tomography scan with oral contrast of the neck or chest. The gold standard for diagnosis includes a fluoroscopic contrast esophagram using gastrografin followed by thin barium if the diagnosis is not confirmed (**Fig. 2**). Esophagogastroduodenoscopy is useful to determine the extent of esophageal or conduit necrosis, especially in patients with postesophagectomy leaks or caustic injury.

## GRADING SEVERITY

In 2009, Dr Luketich and colleagues from Pittsburgh developed a score, the Pittsburgh Severity Score (PSS), based on a set of clinical variables intended to predict patient outcomes and guide clinical management. The scoring system includes advanced age, tachycardia, leukocytosis, presence of pleural

effusion, fever, presence of a noncontained leak, respiratory compromise, extended time to diagnosis, presence of cancer, and hypotension. Each variable is assigned 1 to 3 points, and a maximum score is 18. Mortality was found to be 100% in patients with a score of 9 or greater.[5]

Multiple retrospective studies have sought to validate the usefulness of the PSS. In the largest of these studies, 288 patients with spontaneous, traumatic, and iatrogenic esophageal perforations across 11 countries were evaluated and grouped based on their PSS. Mean PSS was 5.8. PSS was significantly higher in patients who ultimately expired and in patients who required operative management. PSS greater than 5 was associated with increased morbidity, increased length of stay, operative intervention, and mortality. Mortality rate increased by 8 times when compared with the patients with a PSS of 3 to 4 and 18 times when compared with patients with a PSS of 2 or less.[6] A more recent albeit smaller (73 patients) case series again sought to validate the usefulness of the PSS. This series showed that higher PSS was associated with intensive care unit (ICU) admission, longer hospital length of stay, operative intervention, operative reintervention, postperforation complications, and mortality.[7]

## MANAGEMENT

Once the diagnosis of esophageal perforation is confirmed, the patient should be immediately stabilized with proper resuscitation including large-bore intravenous (IV) catheters and IV fluid bolus with isotonic crystalloid. The patient should be made strictly NPO. Broad spectrum antibiotics

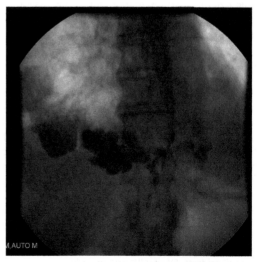

M,AUTO M

**Fig. 2.** An esophagram of an uncontained esophageal perforation.

should be started to cover aerobes and anaerobes, with consideration of antifungal therapy, especially in patients who have been on long-term proton pump inhibitor therapy or immunosuppression.[8] The remainder of management will depend on cause and location of perforation and extent of mediastinal and pleural contamination but should focus on controlling the perforation, restoring luminal integrity, and removing and debriding all extraluminal contamination as necessary.

## Surgical Options for Management

Multiple different surgical interventions have been described for treating esophageal perforation. Primary repair is possible in many settings but is contraindicated in diffuse mediastinal necrosis, a large perforation unable to be reapproximated, esophageal malignancy, preexisting end-stage benign esophageal disease (ie, achalasia), and clinical instability.[9–11] Primary repair involves identifying the site of perforation, opening the muscle layer to expose the full mucosal defect, and repairing the esophagus in 2 layers. The site is often buttressed with a well-vascularized muscle flap, omental flap, or pleural flap to aid in healing. Cervical drainage remains the surgical intervention of choice for cervical perforations and includes exposing the site of perforation and leaving surgical drains (ie, penrose drains) in the contaminated field, with the option to buttress the area with a well-vascularized muscle flap. If a patient is unable to tolerate extensive surgery, a T-tube can be placed, creating a controlled fistula. Esophageal diversion may be necessary in the setting of an unstable patient, if repair is not possible due to the size of the defect or friability of the surrounding tissue or preexisting esophageal disease including untreated achalasia, and undilatable stricture, or malignancy. Diversion includes washing out and debriding any mediastinal or pleural contamination, diversion via a cervical esophagostomy, resecting the remaining esophagus, placing a gastric tube for venting, and placing a jejunostomy tube for feeding. In addition to the aforementioned surgical options, hybrid approaches have been described. These mainly include surgical washout of any contamination and fully covered stent placement for perforation control. Mortality rate with surgical intervention ranges from 6% to 39% depending on the site of perforation, severity, and length of time to diagnosis.[2,12]

Recently, a shift toward less aggressive surgical intervention has been described. In a recent publication by Chu and colleagues, a 6-step algorithm outlining surgical management in esophageal perforation was described. The straight forward steps were designed for surgeons without a high level of expertise and can be performed by most centers without the need for transfer to a specialized facility. Their case series performing these steps, which essentially included 14 days of esophageal exclusion, resulted in one mortality from advanced cirrhosis but otherwise had a 100% resolution of sepsis rate and all patients were able to return to a regular diet.[13] Esophageal exclusion in these cases was performed with a 0-chromic at the cervical esophagus and a 0-chromic at the abdominal esophagus.[13] In addition, a article by Millan and colleagues described an algorithm for damage control for esophageal injuries from trauma, which recommends primary repair, nasogastric tube placement, and close postoperative care in the ICU. They recommend the "Less is Better" philosophy, which includes avoidance of cervical esophagostomies.[14] Traditional surgical approaches to esophageal perforation require a thoracotomy for access and repair in an already sick patient. A thoracotomy is associated with a higher rate of respiratory complications and can take a substantial amount of time to perform and close. Given these disadvantages, there is an interest in shifting to less invasive and even nonsurgical options to close perforations.

## Endoscopic Management

Multiple endoscopic interventions to treat esophageal perforation have been described including self-expanding, removable metal stent placement, endoscopic clipping, and endovac therapy. Stent placement is the most widely described, especially with a hybrid surgical approach; however, stent migration and malpositioning are possible especially when used in close proximity to the gastroesophageal junction. Risk factors associated with stent failure include injury in the proximal cervical esophagus, injury that transverses the gastroesophageal junction, length of injury longer than 6 cm, and anastomotic leak associated with a more distal conduit leak.[15] Endoscopic clipping either over-the-scope or through-the-scope has been described most successfully in patients with small defects, healthy compliant surrounding tissue, and mucosa that can be approximated with minimal tension. This technique is used most frequently in iatrogenic injuries with minimal extraluminal contamination. In addition, endoscopic suturing can be used in the same clinical settings.[16] Endovac therapy has been successfully described for smaller defects with more contained contamination and in patients who cannot tolerate more invasive procedures. The endovac therapy requires maintaining the device via a nasogastric tube for potentially weeks at a time and requires invasive regular device changes.[17] Endoscopic management can have 100% survival with careful patient selection, including early diagnosis, evidence of contained perforations, and limited extraluminal soilage.[18–20] Endoscopic management of the perforation is often done in conjunction with a video-assisted thoracoscopic surgery or minimally invasive drainage of the pleural space to prevent on-going sepsis.

### Stenting

Multiple recent case series describe results with endoscopic stent placement in a variety of patient populations; however, no randomized controlled trials exist to compare it with the previous gold standard of surgical intervention. A 2017 systematic review found that stent placement and conservative management has become increasingly used, but the effects on mortality remain unclear.[21] A retrospective case review including 142 consecutive patients over a 25-year time period showed 23% of patients received stents compared with surgical intervention for 77%. Stents were more frequently used for malignant perforations. Twenty percent of patients who underwent surgical repair required reintervention including both stent or surgery. Sixty-seven percent of stent patients healed their injury after a single stent, and another 8% healed after an endoscopic stent reposition. Stents placed at the gastroesophageal junction were more likely to fail than stents placed into the thoracic esophagus.[22]

Two case series including 76 and 77 patients looked at patients who only underwent stent placement for perforations due to anastomotic leak, fistulae, iatrogenic injuries, and primary perforations. These series describe a 100% technical success with stent placement. Successful esophageal closure was reported in 89% and 74% of patients. Median length of ICU stay was 3 days and hospital stay was 10 days. Described complications included prolonged intubation, stent migration, dysphagia, and aspiration pneumonia. Factors associated with successful primary esophageal closure included a shorter time between diagnosis and stent placement and a smaller luminal opening size.[23,24] In addition, a recent systematic review describing stent experience in anastomotic leaks and benign perforations included 1752 patients across 66 studies. Technical and clinical success rates were 96% and 87%. Stent migration rate was reported at 12%, and reintervention rate was reported at 20%. Mortality rate was 7%, with poststent hospital length of stay ranging from 5 to 67 days. Plastic stents were associated with higher migration rates, higher repositioning rates, and lower technical success rates than metallic stents. Specifically in the anastomotic leak patients, plastic stents were associated with higher perforation rates than metallic stents. The only long-term complication reported was stricture and was observed in 2% of patients.[25,26]

Stent placement in the trauma population has also been described. Mubang and colleagues suggest nonoperative management should be considered in trauma patients who have a contained leak, are mildly symptomatic, and have minimal evidence of clinical sepsis. In the patients who meet this criterium, conservative management with stent placement was associated with lower cost, fewer ICU days, shorter hospitalization, quicker resumption of oral intake, and equivalent overall mortality when compared with surgical interventions.[27]

Endoscopic suturing as an adjunct to esophageal stenting has been suggested to improve primary repair rate. A retrospective case review including 114 patients describes this technique; however, overall outcomes were not improved. Similar defect repair rates between the combined endoscopic suturing and stent group when compared with the stent alone group were realized. In addition, the time to defect closure, migration rate, time to migration, and rate of additional stent requirement were all not statistically different between groups. Procedure time, however, was significantly longer, nearly double, in the endoscopic suturing group.[28]

### Endoscopic Vacuum Therapy

Endoscopic vacuum therapy (EVT) was first described for use in the upper gastrointestinal (GI) tract in 2008 and since that time has grown in popularity. The endo sponge is placed via an over tube and can be placed transmurally within the cavity (intracavitary) or overlying the defect while remaining inside of the GI tract (intraluminal). This decision is made primarily based on perforation and cavity size, but is operator dependent. The free end of the sponge device is then pulled through the nose for connection to a suction canister. Sponges and sponge placement kits are commercially available. Multiple small series case reports exist outlining the indications, efficacy, and safety profile of these devices. Continuous suction promotes healing by apposition of the wound edges, granulation of healthy tissue, neovascularization, control of the septic focus through active drainage, and diversion of secretions. The most severe complication described is major bleeding. Additional minor complications include posttreatment stricture formation, dislodgement, and minor bleeding.[17] Sponge placement can be performed in either the GI laboratory or the operating room, with the operating room associated with a significantly higher cost but shorter overall procedure time. Provider proficiency is typically achieved after an average of 10 cases.[29]

An early case series of postoperative leak patients described an 86% defect closure rate with a median duration of endovac treatment of 13 days. Early and rapid control of sepsis was described with most patients not requiring sponge replacement.[30] When placed for refractory cervical, thoracic, or gastric conduit leaks, defined as continued leak after failure of another conservative treatment, complete healing was achieved in 63% of patients. Patients required a median of 5 procedures and a median treatment duration of 19 days. No major adverse events were reported.[31] Although originally described for postoperative leaks, indication for EVT has expanded to acute esophageal perforation. A recent case series describes its use in the upper, middle, and lower esophagus for spontaneous and iatrogenic perforations. All patients had successful closure of their perforation with no adverse events or complications. Median treatment duration was 7.5 days and median number of sponge exchanges was 2.5.[32] A systematic review comparing EVT with stenting for all indications showed superiority of EVT in multiple categories including a higher closure rate, a lower mortality rate, a shorter treatment duration, and a lower posttherapy stricture rate.[17]

A new device combining both EVT and self-expanding metal stents was recently developed and is undergoing clinical trials. VACStent (VAC-Stent Medtec AG, Switzerland) combines a dumbbell-shaped fully covered 72 mm long stent with a continuous suction sponge. The shape was developed to prevent stent migration and is currently only available in one size. Early case series describing its use in postoperative leaks as well as iatrogenic and spontaneous perforation show a clinical success rate of 60% with a median duration of treatment of 4.8 days. Technical success of device placement was 100%. Of note, any attempt at enteral feedings resulted in clogging of the suction portion of the device.[33]

## World Society of Emergency Surgery Guidelines

The World Society of Emergency Surgery published guidelines pertaining to operative versus nonoperative candidacy after its fifth congress, which met in June of 2018. Those guidelines are summarized here:

Criteria for nonoperative management of esophageal perforations:

- Delay in management of less than 24 hours
- Absence of signs and symptoms of sepsis
- Cervical or thoracic location of the esophageal perforation
- Contained perforation, with minimal periesophageal extravasation of contrast material and intraesophageal drainage
- Absence of massive pleural contamination
- No preexistent esophageal disease
- Possibility of close surveillance by an expert esophageal team
- Availability of round-the-clock surgical and radiological skills

Criteria for operative management of esophageal perforations:

- Surgery should be undertaken in all patients who do not meet nonoperative criteria
- Patients should be taken to the operating room as soon as possible
- Repair of esophageal perforations via a minimally invasive technique should be considered[34]

Although operative management is still recommended, what operative management entails is changing. The days of requiring a thoracotomy for all esophageal perforations is gone. The perforation itself can be addressed endoscopically in most of the cases. Surgery, particularly minimally invasive surgery, is useful for draining the chest and mediastinum from contamination.

## SUMMARY

Esophageal perforation is a rare but potentially fatal disease process that requires prompt diagnosis and treatment. Surgery has historically been required for the treatment of these patients but a shift toward endoscopic therapies has occurred. Although no randomized controlled trials exist to compare patient outcomes, many case series and systematic analyses describe their indications, efficacy, and safety profile. Endoscopic stenting and endoscopic vacuum therapy are the 2 therapies most widely described across a diverse patient population and seem to be safe and effective when treating esophageal perforation, in the proper clinical setting. Guidelines and scoring systems exist to help direct management and stratify patient risk.

## CLINICS CARE POINTS

- Esophageal perforation is a rare but severe disease process that requires prompt diagnosis and treatment.
- Initial management includes resuscitation, broad spectrum antibiotics, consideration of antifungal therapy, controlling the perforation, restoring luminal integrity, and debriding all extraluminal contamination.
- Surgical intervention has historically been the mainstay of treatment; however, a shift toward endoscopic treatment exists, despite no randomized clinical trials comparing patient outcomes.
- Self-expanding metal stents and endoscopic vacuum therapy have been widely described across a diverse patient population and seem to be safe and effective as a treatment strategy, in the proper clinical setting.
- For patients who are hemodynamically unstable or show signs of clinical deterioration, operative debridement and control of contamination is recommended.
- In hemodynamically stable patients with evidence of esophageal perforation, endovac or stent placement may be an appropriate treatment.
- All patients with suspicion of esophageal perforation should be started on appropriate antimicrobial therapy.

## DISCLOSURES

K. Fairbairn has nothing to disclose. S.G. Worrell is a consultant for Intuitive and Bristol Meyer Squibs.

## REFERENCES

1. Vidarsdottir H, Blondal S, Alfredsson H, et al. Oesophageal perforations in iceland: a whole population study on incidence, aetiology and surgical outcome. Thorac Cardiovasc Surg 2010;58(8):476–80.
2. Brinster CJ, Singhal S, Lee L, et al. Evolving options in the management of esophageal perforation. Ann Thorac Surg 2004;77:1475.
3. Shaker H, Elsayed H, Whittle I, et al. The influence of the 'golden 24-h rule' on the prognosis of oesophageal perforation in the modern era. Eur J Cardio Thorac Surg 2010;38:216.
4. Vallböhmer D, Hölscher AH, Hölscher M, et al. Options in the management of esophageal perforation: analysis over a 12-year period. Dis Esophagus 2010;23:185.
5. Abbas G, Schuchert MJ, Pettiford BL, et al. Contemporaneous management of esophageal perforation. Surgery 2009;146(4):749–55.
6. Schweigert M, Sousa HS, Solymosi N, et al. Spotlight on esophageal perforation: a multinational study using the Pittsburgh esophageal perforation severity scoring system. J Thorac Cardiovasc Surg 2016 Apr;151(4):1002–9.
7. Moletta L, Pierobon ES, Capovilla G, et al. Could the Pittsburgh Severity Score guide the treatment of esophageal perforation? Experience of a single referral center. J Trauma Acute Care Surg 2022;92(1):108–16.
8. DeVivo A, Sheng AY, Koyfman A, et al. High risk and low prevalence diseases: esophageal perforation. Am J Emerg Med 2022;53:29–36.
9. Salo JA, Isolauri JO, Heikkila LJ, et al. Management of delayed esophageal perforation with mediastinal sepsis. Esophagectomy or primary repair? J Thorac Cardiovasc Surg 1993;106:1088.
10. Kim-Deobald J, Kozarek RA. Esophageal perforation: an 8-year review of a multispecialty clinic's experience. Am J Gastroenterol 1992;87:1112.
11. Wright CD, Mathisen DJ, Wain JC, et al. Reinforced primary repair of the thoracic esophageal perforation. Ann Thorac Surg 1995;60:245.
12. Jones WG 2nd, Ginsberg RJ. Esophageal perforation: a continuing challenge. Ann Thorac Surg 1992;53:534.
13. Chu QD, Candal R, White RK. A novel and simple method of managing thoracic esophageal perforation: the "ASSIST" approach. Am Surg 2021;0(0):1–4.
14. Millan M, Parra MW, Sanchez-Restepo B. Primary repair: damage control surgery in esophageal trauma. Colomb Méd 2021;52(2):e4094806.
15. Freeman RK, Ascioti AJ, Giannini T, et al. Analysis of unsuccessful esophageal stent placements for esophageal perforation, fistula, or anastomotic leak. Ann Thorac Surg 2012;94:959.
16. Barakat MT, Girotra M, Banerjee S. (Re)building the wall: recurrent boerhaave syndrome managed by over-the-scope clip and covered metallic stent placement. Dig Dis Sci 2018;63:1139.
17. Livingstone I, Pollock L, Sgromo B, et al. Current status of endoscopic vacuum therapy in the management of esophageal perforations and post-operative leaks. Clin Endosc 2021 Nov;54(6):787–97.
18. Altorjay A, Kiss J, Vörös A, et al. Nonoperative management of esophageal perforations. Is it justified? Ann Surg 1997;225:415.
19. Cameron JL, Kieffer RF, Hendrix TR, et al. Selective nonoperative management of contained intrathoracic esophageal disruptions. Ann Thorac Surg 1979;27:404.
20. Vogel SB, Rout WR, Martin TD, et al. Esophageal perforation in adults: aggressive, conservative treatment lowers morbidity and mortality. Ann Surg 2005; 241:1016.

21. Sdralis EIK, Petousis S, Rashid F, et al. Epidemiology, diagnosis, and management of esophageal perforations: systematic review. Dis Esophagus 2017;30(8):1–6.
22. Axtell AL, Gaissert HA, Morse CR, et al. Management and outcomes of esophageal perforation. Dis Esophagus 2022;35(1):doab039.
23. El Hajj I, Imperiale T, Rex D, et al. Treatment of esophageal leaks, fistulae, and perforations with temporary stents: evaluation of efficacy, adverse events, and factors associated with successful outcomes. Gastrointest Endosc 2014;79(4):589–98.
24. Ben-David K, Behrns K, Hochwald S, et al. Esophageal perforation management using a multidisciplinary minimally invasive treatment algorithm. J Am Coll Surg 2014;218(4):768–74.
25. Kamarajah S, Bundred J, Spence G, et al. Critical appraisal of the impact of oesophageal stents in the management of oesophageal anastomotic leaks and benign oesophageal perforations: an updated systematic review. World J Surg 2020;44:1173–89.
26. Lange B, Demirakca S, Kahler G, et al. Experience with fully covered self-expandable metal stents for esophageal leakage in children. Klin Pädiatr 2020; 232(01):13–9.
27. Mubang RN, Sigmon DF, Stawicki SP. Esophageal trauma. Treasure Island (FL): StatPearls Publishing; 2022. StatPearls [Internet].
28. Obaitan I, DeWitt JM, Bick BL, et al. The addition of fexible endoscopic suturing to stenting for the management of transmural esophageal wall defects: a single tertiary center experience. Surg Endosc 2021;35(11):6379–89.
29. Ward MA, Hassan T, Burdick JS, et al. Endoscopic vacuum assisted wound closure (EVAC) device to treat esophageal and gastric leaks: assessing time to proficiency and cost. Surg Endosc 2019;33(12): 3970–5.
30. Mastoridis S, Chana P, Singh M, et al. Endoscopic vacuum therapy (EVT) in the management of oesophageal perforations and post-operative leaks. Minim Invasive Ther Allied Technol 2022;31(3): 380–8.
31. De Pasqual CA, Mengardo V, Tomba F, et al. Effectiveness of endoscopic vacuum therapy as rescue treatment in refractory leaks after gastroesophageal surgery. Updates Surg 2021;73(2): 607–14.
32. Stathopoulos P, Zumblick M, Wächter S, et al. Endoscopic vacuum therapy (EVT) for acute esophageal perforation: Could it replace surgery? Endosc Int Open 2022;10(5):E686–93.
33. Chon SH, Scherdel J, Rieck I, et al. A new hybrid stent using endoscopic vacuum therapy in treating esophageal leaks: a prospective single-center experience of its safety and feasibility with midterm follow-up. Dis Esophagus 2022;35(4):doab067.
34. Chirica M, Kelly MD, Siboni S, et al. Esophageal emergencies: WSES guidelines. World J Emerg Surg 2019;14:26.

# Gastroesophageal Reflux Disease in 2023
## When to Operate and Current Endoscopic Options for Antireflux Therapy

Anuj Shah, MD[a], Min P. Kim, MD[b],*

**KEYWORDS**

- Transoral incisionless fundoplication • TIF • RFA • Radiofrequency ablation

**KEY POINTS**

- Patients with medically refractory gastroesophageal reflux disease (GERD) should undergo endoscopy and esophagram with possible manometry, 24-h impedance, or BRAVO to determine if surgical endoscopic procedure could improve patient's symptoms.
- Surgical fundoplication has better long-term outcomes compared with endoscopic procedures for the treatment of medically refractory GERD with or without hiatal hernia.
- Endoscopic procedure (radiofrequency ablation) and transoral incisionless fundoplication provide improved outcomes compared with medical therapy for patients with medically refractory GERD with no hiatal hernia of hiatal hernia <3 cm.

## INTRODUCTION

Gastroesophageal reflux disease (GERD) is the most common gastrointestinal (GI) disorder in the United States. It has a prevalence of 18% to 27% in the United States.[1] GERD is defined by the reflux of gastric contents from the stomach into the esophagus. The mechanisms of GERD can be intrinsic, structural, or both. GERD symptoms are usually divided into typical (classic esophageal) and atypical (extraesophageal) symptoms. The typical symptoms are heartburn, regurgitation, or chest pain felt by the patient when acid or bile irritates the esophageal mucosa. The atypical symptoms are cough or sore through when the acid or nonacid irritates the larynx, pharynx, or aspirates in the pulmonary system.[2,3] This array of symptoms has been shown to significantly impact the quality of life.[4] Although there is no known cause to explain the development of GERD, there are several risk factors that have been associated with GERD, such as older age, male sex, race, intake of analgesics, consumption of certain types of foods and drinks, smoking, high body mass index (BMI).

Moreover, motor abnormalities such as esophageal dysmotility, causing impaired esophageal acid clearance, dysfunctional lower esophageal sphincter (LES), and delayed gastric emptying can contribute to GERD. The mainstay of treatment is lifestyle changes and medical management. Further testing is needed when patients have symptoms despite medical therapy. In this article, we discuss diagnosing and treating patients with GERD.

### Epidemiology

The prevalence of GERD is approximately 18% to 27% in the United States.[5] The incidence of GERD

a Department of Surgery, Houston Methodist Hospital, 6550 Fannin St SM1661, Houston, TX 77030, USA;
b Division of Thoracic Surgery, Department of Surgery, Houston Methodist Hospital, 6550 Fannin St SM1661, Houston, TX 77030, USA
* Corresponding author.
*E-mail address:* mpkim@houstonmethodist.org
Twitter: @DrMinPKim (M.P.K.)

Thorac Surg Clin 33 (2023) 125–134
https://doi.org/10.1016/j.thorsurg.2023.01.010

in the western world was approximately 5 per 1000 person-years or 0.5% per year. Epidemiologic estimates for the prevalence of GERD are limited as they are based on the assumption that symptoms are the only indicators of GERD. The severity of symptoms and severity of disease does not correlate in patients. More women present with GERD symptoms, but men seem to have a more severe disease on endoscopy with a higher incidence of Barrett's esophagus (BE).[6–8]

## Pathophysiology

Three factors cause gastroesophageal reflux the tone of the LES, esophageal motility, and the presence of a hiatal hernia. First, the abnormal tone of LES causes GERD. The LES maintains pressures greater than the intra-gastric pressures with transient relaxation stimulated by food intake. Patients with symptoms of GERD, however, have been noted to have a more frequent episode of relaxation of the LES. These relaxations account for 48% to 72% of GERD symptoms.[9] Smoking, alcohol intake, pregnancy, obesity, caffeine, and medications have also been found to affect the tone of the LES. Second, impaired esophageal motility may play a role in GERD.[10] The esophageal motility plays a role in clearing refluxed contents from the esophagus. Diener and colleagues[11] found that 21% of patients with GERD had impaired esophageal peristalsis, and the resulting decreased clearance of reflux contacts was related to severe GERD symptoms. Finally, the presence of a hiatal hernia is associated with worsening GERD symptoms. Although hiatal hernia and GERD are independent diagnoses, it has been shown that the presence of a hiatal hernia does worsen GERD symptoms. It is important to note that in the literature, it has been found that small sliding hiatal hernias had similar LES function abnormalities compared with patients with GERD but without hiatal hernia. However, patients with large hiatal hernia and GERD were noted to have shorter and weaker LES. These patients also had a more severe degree of esophagitis.[12]

## Initial Diagnosis

The evaluation of patients with GERD will start by obtaining a careful history. The patient should be asked about heartburn and if the symptoms are related to the position, diet, and its impact on sleep. In addition, one should ask about dysphagia and bloating, both symptoms that surgeons think about typically after surgery, but understanding their degree of dysphagia and bloating before surgery provides surgeons context to evaluate these

symptoms after surgery. Finally, the patient should be asked about using medications to treat reflux. In addition to the questions related to typical symptoms, patients should be asked about atypical symptoms. Patients should be asked if they have a voice change or a bitter taste in their mouth and if they have a cough and a history of pneumonia. All of this helps to determine if the patient has typical and atypical symptoms as their main symptoms associated with GERD. GERD diagnoses are typically made based on these symptoms. The first-line treatment for most of these patients is generally lifestyle modification and medical management.

## Lifestyle Changes and Medical Management

Lifestyle modifications, including weight loss and elevation of the head of the bed, are known to be effective in the management of GERD. Diet modification is controversial and not routinely recommended per the guidelines published by the American College of Gastroenterology.[13] If these modifications are ineffective, patients are usually started on empiric proton pump inhibitors (PPIs), and response to this treatment would confirm the diagnosis of GERD. Other medical therapy includes antacids and antisecretory agents such as H2 histamine receptor antagonists. Of these options, PPI is considered the most effective for symptom control, healing of underlying esophagitis, and decreased relapse rates compared with H2 histamine receptor blockers.[14,15] Generally, PPIs are started at a standard dose once daily for a period of 8 weeks and have been shown to heal esophagitis in 86% of the patients.[16,17] However, there has been mounting evidence regarding the long-term side effects of PPI use, including increased risk of osteoporosis,[18] gastric cancer, and respiratory and urinary infections.[19,20]

## Medically Refractory Gastroesophageal Reflux Disease

In patients with symptoms despite lifestyle modification, further studies are needed to categorize the degree of GERD and determine the optimal treatment for the patient. Endoscopy is a good test to characterize the extent of GERD. GERD is classified into three categories based on the endoscopic and histopathologic appearance of the mucosa. First, non-erosive reflux disease (NRE) is endoscopy-negative reflux disease characterized by GERD symptoms without esophageal injuries, constituting 60% to 70% of reflux disease. Second, erosive esophagitis (EE): This is characterized by visible breaks in the distal esophageal mucosa with or without symptoms of GERD, which constitute 30%. Finally, BE is a histopathologic diagnosis. The distal esophageal mucosa, normally lined by stratified squamous epithelium, changes to the metaplastic columnar epithelium, which constitutes 6% to 12% of reflux disease. According to the Lyon consensus, three endoscopic findings diagnose pathologic gastro-esophageal reflux.[21] The presence of Los Angeles (LA) grade C or D EE, BE, and peptic stricture. These three endoscopic criteria provide conclusive evidence for pathologic reflux and patients do not need additional diagnostic studies to support the diagnosis of GERD. The endoscopy can also show the presence of a hiatal hernia. Patients with pathologic GERD with no hiatal hernia or sliding hiatal hernia should undergo manometry.

In the group of patients with small or no hiatal hernia, the manometry could help determine optimal endoscopic or minimally invasive surgical therapy for the patient. Patients with poor motility should undergo minimally invasive hiatal hernia repair with partial fundoplication. Manometry also provided information on if the patient had disorders of EGD outflow such as Achalasia or esophagogastric junction outflow obstruction (EGJOO) or disorders of peristalsis such as absent contractility, distal esophageal spasm, hypercontractile esophagus, or ineffective esophageal motility using the Chicago Classification version 4.[22] Based on the findings, we would perform appropriate operations.

The diagnosis of hiatal hernia can be further confirmed on a timed barium study with barium liquid and tablet. The study can provide information about the presence of the hiatal hernia and its size. If the patient has a type II, III, or IV hiatal hernia with reflux, the patient should undergo minimally invasive hiatal hernia repair with fundoplication. None of the endoscopic GERD therapy is designed to treat patients with type II, III, or IV hiatal hernia.

If the patient has no structural abnormality on the esophagram and no abnormalities on endoscopy, the patient should undergo an impedance 24-h pH test. The test measures the presence of acid or nonacid reflux and provides information about the correlation of symptoms with the reflux event. The Lyon consensus statement showed that the acid exposure time (AET) in the impedance 24-h pH test is the most reproducible and reliable marker for the diagnosis of reflux.[21] If the patient has > 6% AET, it provides a diagnosis of reflux, and if the AET is < 4%, the acid exposure is normal. The study is inconclusive if the AET is 4% to 6%. At this point, the next dataset we look at is the number of reflux episodes in 24 h. If the number is > 80, it is an abnormal study consistent with reflux; if it is < 40, it is normal; if it is between 40 and 80 events, the study is inconclusive.[23] In addition to these criteria, as surgeons, we look at the DeMeester score. The DeMeester Score is a composite score using the AET and the total number of reflux as well as the number of episodes > 5 min and longest episode in minutes, and percent of the upright time in reflux with a score > 14.72 is abnormal.[24] If the patient has any abnormal score, the patient should be considered for endoscopic or minimally invasive treatment of GERD. Furthermore, symptom correlation in the 24-h impedance test is helpful in patients with atypical GERD symptoms such as cough, throat clearing, globus sensation, and asthma. The symptom association probability can help to determine if atypical GERD symptoms are related to acid or nonacid reflux. The outcomes for treatment of atypical GERD symptoms are not as good as the relief of typical symptoms, likely because atypical could be from the GI or non-GI source (allergies, asthma, bronchitis, postnasal drip) or both.[25] Thus, relief from the GI source could be improved with surgery, but if the symptom is related to non-GI or a combination of GI and non-GI sources, the symptoms may not resolve completely. Thus, if there is a good symptom association probability, there is a good chance the atypical symptoms will resolve with surgical intervention.

Lastly, if the patient has normal esophageal, normal endoscopy, and 24-h pH impedance study, we typically send the patient for a 48-h BRAVO test. The advantage of this test is it provides a longer time frame to see if the acid reflux is related to symptoms. The disadvantage of this test is that it only picks up acid-related events. Although 24-h pH impedance detects both acid and non-acid reflux and provides the complete picture, the BRAVO is designed to evaluate acid reflux only. Thus, we use the BRAVO and second-line test. If this test is normal, we would consider the patient to have non-ulcer dyspepsia[26] defined as persistent or recurrent abdominal pain or abdominal discomfort in the upper abdomen without abnormality on the diagnostic test. Typically, there is no correlation between symptoms and findings. We tell patients that surgical intervention at the gastroesophageal junction will not improve their symptoms and recommend further workup to determine the potential source. We would work with our gastroenterology colleagues on checking for H pylori, CT of the abdomen, the US of the abdomen, and gastric emptying study to fully evaluate the abdomen and treat it based on the finding. If there are still no obvious abnormalities, a trial of PPI, prokinetics, sucralfate, anticholinergics, and low-dose antidepressants have been used to manage this group of patients.

### Endoscopic Options: Sliding Hiatal Hernia and Normal Motility with Pathologic Gastroesophageal Reflux Disease

Patients with a small sliding hiatal hernia (<3 cm) or no hiatal hernia with normal motility and pathologic GERD will have the best outcome with MSA or surgical fundoplication. Patients who are not interested in surgical treatment should consider endoscopic options. Two endoscopic options are STRETTA and TIF procedure.

### Endoscopic Therapy for Gastroesophageal Reflux Disease

Surgical intervention remains the gold standard for the treatment of GERD. However, if a patient does not want to undergo surgery, there are two endoscopic options: STRETTA using radiofrequency ablation and TIF creating endoscopic fundoplication.

## STRETTA: RADIOFREQUENCY ABLATION
### Introduction

The STRETTA system (Mederi Therapeutics, Norwalk, CT, USA) used radiofrequency ablation technology to augment the LES. The system uses radiofrequency energy via a balloon catheter on the LES muscle and gastric cardia. Although the mechanism of action is not fully understood, the proposed mechanism is the hypertrophy of the muscularis propria and reduced transient LES relaxation after RFA.[27,28]

The STRETTA system (Mederi Therapeutics, Norwalk, CT, USA) was approved by the FDA in 2000. The system typically delivers low-power (5 W) energy with a thermocouple that ensures avoidance of high temperatures at muscularis (>85°C) and mucosal levels (>50°C).

### Preoperative Planning and Indications

The ideal candidates for STRETTA, according to the Society of American Gastrointestinal and Endoscopic Surgeons, are 18 years or older patients with symptoms >6 months, who are partially or completely responsive to medical therapy and have the following characteristics.

1. Symptoms: Frequent heartburn and/or regurgitation
2. Medically refractory: Unsatisfactory control of symptoms with high-dose PPIs
3. Esophagram: No hiatal hernia or hiatal hernia < 3 cm.

4. Manometry: Adequate esophageal peristalsis and normal LES relaxation.
5. 24-h pH study: Abnormal DeMeester score >14.7 with total acid exposure time >4%

### Contraindication for STRETTA

1. Symptoms: significant dysphagia
2. Endoscopy: Savary–Miller Grade III or Grade IV esophagitis
3. Manometry: inadequate peristalsis and incomplete LES relaxation in response to a swallow

### Prep and Patient Positioning

Patients are placed in either left lateral decubitus or supine position with conscious sedation for the procedure.

Steps of STRETTA procedure (**Fig. 1**) are as follows:

1. Endoscopy is performed to ensure that there is no contraindication for the procedure.
2. Distance from incisors to the squamocolumnar junction is measured.
3. An endoscope is removed, and an RFA catheter is passed transorally and placed 2 cm above the measured Z-Line.
4. Four-needle electrodes are deployed to a preset length of 5.5 mm, and RFA is initiated.
5. Each electrode delivers 90 s of RFA to achieve a target temperature of 85° Celsius.
6. Additional lesions are made by rotating and changing the linear position of the catheter to make several rings 2 cm above and below the cardia of the stomach
7. After this, the RFA catheter is removed
8. Endoscopy is performed to ensure no adverse effect of the RFA.

### Recovery and Rehabilitation

Patients are generally able to return to work the next day. For the first 3 days after the procedure, patients will usually follow a modified diet and slowly advanced diet.

### Outcomes

Multiple RCTs and systematic reviews have shown the benefits and Efficacy of RFA. In the long-term follow-up study, 72% of patients normalized their GERD-health-related quality of life (GERD-HRQL) score, and 64% of patients reduced PPI use by 50% or more at the 10-year mark.[29] Very few studies compare the STRETTA to laparoscopic fundoplication, and none of the studies is a multicenter randomized controlled trial to provide the best evidence between the groups. A retrospective cohort study compared laparoscopic Toupet

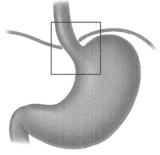

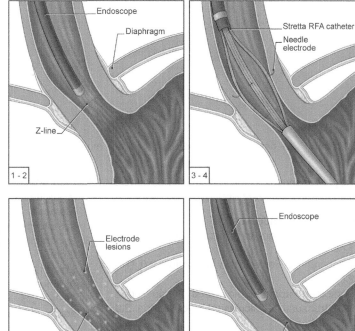

1. Endoscopy is performed to ensure that there is no contraindication for the procedure
2. Distance from incisors to the z-line is measured
3. Endoscope is removed, and an RFA catheter is passed transorally and placed 2 cm above the measured z-line
4. Four-needle electrodes are deployed to a preset length of 5.5mm, and RFA is initiated
5. Each electrode delivers 90 seconds of RFA to achieve a target temperature of 85 °C
6. Additional lesions are made by rotating and changing the linear position of the catheter to make several rings 2 cm above and below the cardia of the stomach
7. RFA catheter is removed
8. Endoscopy is performed to ensure no adverse effect of the RFA

**Fig. 1.** STRETTA procedure. (*From* Restech, Houston, TX.)

fundoplication ($n = 142$) and STRETTA ($n = 88$) showed that both groups had a decrease in the DeMeester score at 1 year, with 1.4% of patients in the STRETTA group with relapse of symptoms vs. 0% in the fundoplication group ($P = .744$).[30] A small prospective cohort study compared the STRETTA procedure ($n = 47$) to laparoscopic Toupet fundoplication ($n = 51$) in patients with medically refractory GERD and found that patients had a similar impact on extraesophageal symptoms but a significantly higher number of patient satisfaction in laparoscopic Toupet fundoplication group compared with the STRETTA group.[31] In another retrospective cohort study, patients who had laparoscopic Nissen fundoplication ($n = 35$) had significantly greater cough improvement compared with patients who had STRETTA ($n = 48$).[32] One analysis of the evidence between STRETTA and laparoscopic fundoplication concluded that laparoscopic fundoplication is more effective than STRETTA for treating pathologic GERD.[33] They found that patients who underwent laparoscopic fundoplication had greater symptom improvement compared with patients who had STRETTA and a significant decrease in the use of PPI at 5 years (91% vs 51%, $P < .001$).

## Summary

STRETTA is a safe option for treating patients with persistent GERD symptoms. Overall, it is not as effective as surgical intervention and limited only to patients with < 3 cm hiatal hernia with normal motility and pathologic GERD. This is a reasonable option for patients not interested in undergoing minimally invasive antireflux surgery.

## TRANSORAL FUNDOPLICATION
### Introduction

Another endoscopic treatment of GERD is transoral incisionless fundoplication. Although STRETTA attempts to improve symptoms using RFA, the goal of TIF is to create a fundoplication using the endoscopic technique. This procedure creates a full-thickness serosa to serosa plication 3 to 5 cm in length and 200° to 300° partial fundoplication. The device used to perform this procedure is the EsophyX device (EndoGastric Solutions, Inc. Redmond, WA). This device underwent multiple iterations, with the latest one being EsophyX Z. Previous versions were the EsophyX2 and the original EsophyX device.

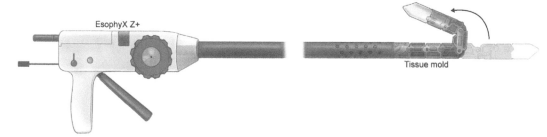

**Fig. 2.** EsophyX Z+ device with a close-up of the tissue mold. (*From* EndoGastric Solutions, Redmond, WA.)

The procedures performed by this device can be divided into four different options. These are.

1. Endoluminal Fundoplication
2. Transoral Incisionless fundoplication 1.0 (TIF 1.0)
3. Transoral Incisionless fundoplication 2.0 (TIF 2.0)
4. Combined laparoscopic hiatal hernia repair with transoral incisionless fundoplication 2.0 (HH-TIF)

The endoluminal fundoplication has evolved with the evolution of the technology of the devices. Stephen Kramer and his team invented the EsophyX device, and he obtained a patent in 2004, and the fasteners for the device were patented in 2009. Using fasteners, the original device was designed to hold and approximate tissue and endoluminal suture the tissue together.

Over time there have been improvements in the fasteners, the endoscopes' accommodation, and the tissue's folding to create the fundoplication.[34] The latest version of the device is the EsophyX Z+ (**Fig. 2**).

TIF 2.0 is performed with or without laparoscopic hiatal hernia repair.[35–39] The TIF 2.0 incorporated a rotational wrap of the cardia and fundus around the distal esophagus, making a 2 to 4-cm length of the wrap over the distal and intra-abdominal esophagus. TIF 2.0 is performed in HH-TIF with laparoscopic hiatal hernia repair with crura closure.

### Preoperative Workup and Indications

The FDA indicates the TIF for treating symptomatic chronic GERD who require and respond to pharmacologic therapy. It is also indicated to narrow the gastroesophageal junction and reduce hiatal hernia =< 2 cm in patients with chronic GERD.

The ideal candidates for TIF are patients with medically refractory symptoms with partially or completely responsive to medical therapy and have the following characteristics.

1. Symptoms: Frequent heartburn and/or regurgitation
2. Medically refractory: Unsatisfactory control of symptoms with high-dose PPIs
3. Esophagram: No hiatal hernia or hiatal hernia < 2 cm.
4. Manometry: Adequate esophageal peristalsis and normal LES relaxation.
5. 24-h pH study: Abnormal DeMeester score >14.7 with total acid exposure time >4

TIF may be performed in patients with hiatal hernias >2 cm if laparoscopic hiatal hernia repair reduces the size to 2 cm or less.

TIF 2.0 Procedure

The patient is positioned supine or left lateral decubitus for TIF 2.0. For HH-TIF, the patient is in the supine position.

### Technique

1. Under general anesthesia, an endoscopy is first performed to visualize the gastroesophageal junction, see the distance of the z-line and gastroesophageal junction from incisors, determine diaphragmatic pinch, and determine if the hiatal hernia is the appropriate size. If HH-TIF is being performed, the endoscopy will ensure adequate repair.
2. Endoscope is then withdrawn, and the EsophyX device is advanced, with the endoscope going through its endoscope channel, as a complex. The endoscope tip extends 10 to 15 cm past the distal tip of the EsophyX device.
3. The complex is advanced into the stomach, and the stomach is insufflated. The endoscope is retroflexed. The complex is advanced until the second blue segment is in the stomach
4. Once in retroflection, to place the EsophyX is placed in a functional position to perform a partial fundoplication, it is rotated to align the back of the tissue mold to the lesser curve. Then endoscope is retracted into the distal

part of the chassis, the tissue mold is closed, and then the endoscope is readvanced through the side hole to retroflex and sees the EsophyX device and GE junction.

5. Once in retroflection, the EsophyX is placed in a functional position to perform a partial fundoplication while taking bites of the proximal stomach at the level of the gastroesophageal junction. This is done by rotating it to align the back of the tissue mold to the lesser curve. An endoscope is retracted into the distal part of the chassis, the tissue mold is closed, and then the endoscope is readvanced through the side hole to retroflex and sees the EsophyX device and GE junction.

6. The helical retractor is advanced until it is in contact with tissue just below the squamocolumnar junction, and it is rotated clockwise to engage the tissue.

7. The entire device is withdrawn to a level where the proximal blue segment is above the GE junction. This sets the device so that the two sharp stylets will exit the device proximal to the blue segment

8. The stomach is deflated, and while doing this, the retractor should be pulled down maximally. This tension will help decide the length of the new valve. Tissue is pulled between the mold and the chassis

9. Once retraction and rotation are done, lock the helical retractor, lock the tissue mold, turn on the invaginator suction, and readvance to the initial length of the GE junction, so stylets do not fire into and through the diaphragm.

10. Fasteners are fired by depressing the safety button and squeezing the trigger.

11. Retractor and mold are unlocked, and the process is repeated for the posterior and anterior corners. Three plications each. Then steps are repeated circumferentially for adequate fixation. No rotation on the greater curve to maximize greater curve length (**Fig. 3**)

## Postoperative Course

Typically, patients go home the same day or on postoperative day 1. Some physicians have patients take antibiotics for the first 2 to 3 days. Patients are asked to take a clear liquid diet for 1 day, then a full liquid diet for 1 week, and then a soft diet without bread and meats. Weightlifting restrictions are usually in place for a few weeks and avoiding vigorous physical activity.

## OUTCOMES

There have been three randomized controlled trials between TIF and high-dose PPI, and all showed favorable results for TIF. The TEMPO randomized control trial compared TIF ($n = 40$) to high-dose PPI ($n = 23$) and found that patients with TIF had a significant reduction of regurgitation

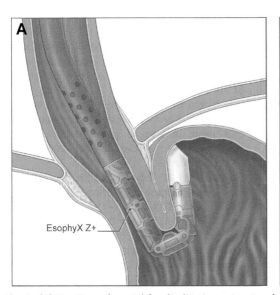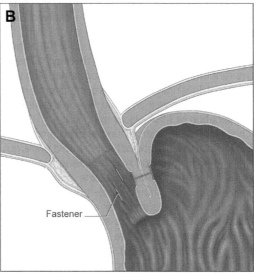

**Fig. 3.** (*A*) Creation of partial fundoplication using EsophyX device. (*B*) Post-procedure appearance of esophagogastric fundoplication proximal to Z line. (*Adapted from* Bell RC, Cadière GB. Transoral rotational esophagogastric fundoplication: technical, anatomical, and safety considerations. Surg Endosc. 2011 Jul;25(7):2387-99. https://doi.org/10.1007/s00464-010-1528-6.)

with 97% in the TIF group vs. 50% in the PPI group (RR 1.9; 95% CI 1.2–3.11, $P = .006$) at 6 months.[40] Moreover, 62% of patients who underwent TIF had eliminated the extraesophageal symptoms compared with 5% in the PPI group (RR 12.9, 95% CI 1.9–88.9, $P = .009$). 90% of patients who had TIF were off of PPI at 6 months. However, there was no significant difference in the normalization of esophageal acid exposure between TIF (54%) and PPIs (52%) at 6 months (RR 1, 95% CI 0.6, 1.7, $P = .914$). Long-term follow-up showed that 66% of patients were off of PPI, 86% of the patients had elimination of the troublesome regurgitation and 80% of patients had resolution of atypical symptoms with TIF at 5 years. The TEMPO trial concluded that TIF 2.0 eliminated regurgitation without significant adverse events or safety concerns. Second, the RESPECT trial[41] was a prospective randomized trial comparing patients undergoing TIF ($n = 45$) or sham endoscopy ($n = 42$). At 6 months, TIF significantly decreased troublesome regurgitation (67%) compared with PPI (45%, $P = .023$). However, at 6 months, both groups had similar improvement in GERD symptoms. The last trial was a randomized double-blinded sham-controlled study[42] with 44 patients in each group. Patients in the TIF procedure had a significantly longer time to remission at 197 days compared with 107 days ($P < .001$). All three showed that TIF had improved symptoms over PPI alone in the short term.

A study looking at the 5-year outcome after TIF ($n = 44$) showed that heartburn was eliminated in 57%, regurgitation was eliminated in 88.2%, and chest pain was eliminated in 83.3%.[43] Another study looking at the 5-year outcome showed that 34% were on daily PPI.[44–46]

At 10 years, 91.7% of patients ($n = 14$) either stopped or halved antisecretory therapy[35] There is no randomized control trial comparing TIF 2.0 to surgical fundoplication. However, overall outcomes are not better than those seen with surgical fundoplication or MSA placement.[37]

Overall, there are a large number of patients with GERD symptoms. These patients should undergo lifestyle modification and medical management. If the patient has symptoms despite conservative therapy, patients should undergo appropriate testing to see if the surgical or endoscopic intervention will improve their symptoms. Minimally invasive fundoplication is the best therapy for patients with pathologic GERD. Patients with small hiatal hernias with normal motility should consider MSA placement. If patients do not want surgical intervention, two endoscopic options are STRETTA and TIF 2.0. Both of them provide e improvement over medical therapy.

## CLINICS CARE POINTS

- Gastroesophageal reflux disease (GERD) has a prevalence of 18% to 27% in the United States
- Mainstay therapy for pathologic GERD is medical management and lifestyle modifications.
- Patients who fail medical management and lifestyle modification should undergo tests including endoscopy, esophagram, manometry, and 24-h impedance test to determine the best surgical or endoscopic intervention.
- Minimally invasive surgical fundoplication is the gold standard for patients with pathologic GERD with or without hiatal hernia.
- Patients with small hiatal hernia with good motility and pathologic GERD who are not interested in fundoplication are good candidates for minimally invasive magnetic sphincter augmentation or endoscopic treatment such as STRETTA or Transoral Incisionless fundoplication 2.0.

## DISCLOSURE

Dr A. Shah has nothing to disclose. Dr M.P. Kim consults for Intuitive Surgical, Medtronic, Olympus, and AstraZeneca.

## REFERENCES

1. El-Serag HB, Sweet S, Winchester CC, et al. Update on the epidemiology of gastro-oesophageal reflux disease: a systematic review. Gut 2014;63(6): 871–80.
2. Vakil N, van Zanten SV, Kahrilas P, et al. The Montreal definition and classification of gastroesophageal reflux disease: a global evidence-based consensus. Am J Gastroenterol 2006;101(8): 1900–20. ; quiz 43.
3. Hom C, Vaezi MF. Extraesophageal manifestations of gastroesophageal reflux disease. Gastroenterol Clin North Am 2013;42(1):71–91.
4. Tack J, Becher A, Mulligan C, et al. Systematic review: the burden of disruptive gastro-oesophageal reflux disease on health-related quality of life. Aliment Pharmacol Ther 2012;35(11):1257–66.
5. Camilleri M, Dubois D, Coulie B, et al. Prevalence and socioeconomic impact of upper gastrointestinal disorders in the United States: results of the US Upper Gastrointestinal Study. Clin Gastroenterol Hepatol 2005;3(6):543–52.

6. Nilsson M, Johnsen R, Ye W, et al. Prevalence of gastro-oesophageal reflux symptoms and the influence of age and sex. Scand J Gastroenterol 2004; 39(11):1040–5.

7. Eusebi LH, Ratnakumaran R, Yuan Y, et al. Global prevalence of, and risk factors for, gastro-oesophageal reflux symptoms: a meta-analysis. Gut 2018;67(3):430–40.

8. Lin M, Gerson LB, Lascar R, et al. Features of gastroesophageal reflux disease in women. Am J Gastroenterol 2004;99(8):1442–7.

9. Mittal RK, McCallum RW. Characteristics and frequency of transient relaxations of the lower esophageal sphincter in patients with reflux esophagitis. Gastroenterology 1988;95(3):593–9.

10. De Giorgi F, Palmiero M, Esposito I, et al. Pathophysiology of gastro-oesophageal reflux disease. Acta Otorhinolaryngol Ital 2006;26(5):241–6.

11. Diener U, Patti MG, Molena D, et al. Esophageal dysmotility and gastroesophageal reflux disease. J Gastrointest Surg 2001;5(3):260–5.

12. Patti MG, Goldberg HI, Arcerito M, et al. Hiatal hernia size affects lower esophageal sphincter function, esophageal acid exposure, and the degree of mucosal injury. Am J Surg 1996;171(1):182–6.

13. Katz PO, Dunbar KB, Schnoll-Sussman FH, et al. ACG Clinical Guideline for the Diagnosis and Management of Gastroesophageal Reflux Disease. Am J Gastroenterol 2022;117(1):27–56.

14. Zhang JX, Ji MY, Song J, et al. Proton pump inhibitor for non-erosive reflux disease: a meta-analysis. World J Gastroenterol 2013;19(45):8408–19.

15. Khan M, Santana J, Donnellan C, et al. Medical treatments in the short term management of reflux oesophagitis. Cochrane Database Syst Rev 2007; 2:CD003244.

16. Wolfe MM, Sachs G. Acid suppression: optimizing therapy for gastroduodenal ulcer healing, gastroesophageal reflux disease, and stress-related erosive syndrome. Gastroenterology 2000;118(2 Suppl 1):S9–31.

17. Hunt R. Acid suppression for reflux disease: "off-the-peg" or a tailored approach? Clin Gastroenterol Hepatol 2012;10(3):210–3.

18. Mizunashi K, Furukawa Y, Katano K, et al. Effect of omeprazole, an inhibitor of H+,K(+)-ATPase, on bone resorption in humans. Calcif Tissue Int 1993; 53(1):21–5.

19. Waldum HL, Sordal O, Fossmark R. Proton pump inhibitors (PPIs) may cause gastric cancer - clinical consequences. Scand J Gastroenterol 2018;53(6):639–42.

20. Koyyada A. Long-term use of proton pump inhibitors as a risk factor for various adverse manifestations. Therapie 2021;76(1):13–21.

21. Gyawali CP, Kahrilas PJ, Savarino E, et al. Modern diagnosis of GERD: the Lyon Consensus. Gut 2018;67(7):1351–62.

22. Yadlapati R, Kahrilas PJ, Fox MR, et al. Esophageal motility disorders on high-resolution manometry: Chicago classification version 4.0((c)). Neuro Gastroenterol Motil 2021;33(1):e14058.

23. Roman S, Gyawali CP, Savarino E, et al. Ambulatory reflux monitoring for diagnosis of gastro-esophageal reflux disease: Update of the Porto consensus and recommendations from an international consensus group. Neuro Gastroenterol Motil 2017; 29(10):1–15.

24. Neto RML, Herbella FAM, Schlottmann F, et al. Does DeMeester score still define GERD? Dis Esophagus 2019;32(5):doy118.

25. So JB, Zeitels SM, Rattner DW. Outcomes of atypical symptoms attributed to gastroesophageal reflux treated by laparoscopic fundoplication. Surgery 1998;124(1):28–32.

26. Locke GR 3rd. Nonulcer dyspepsia: what it is and what it is not. Mayo Clin Proc 1999;74(10):1011–4. quiz 5.

27. Kim MS, Holloway RH, Dent J, et al. Radiofrequency energy delivery to the gastric cardia inhibits triggering of transient lower esophageal sphincter relaxation and gastroesophageal reflux in dogs. Gastrointest Endosc 2003;57(1):17–22.

28. Tam WC, Schoeman MN, Zhang Q, et al. Delivery of radiofrequency energy to the lower oesophageal sphincter and gastric cardia inhibits transient lower oesophageal sphincter relaxations and gastro-oesophageal reflux in patients with reflux disease. Gut 2003;52(4):479–85.

29. Noar M, Squires P, Noar E, et al. Long-term maintenance effect of radiofrequency energy delivery for refractory GERD: a decade later. Surg Endosc 2014;28(8):2323–33.

30. Ma L, Li T, Liu G, et al. STRETTA radiofrequency treatment vs Toupet fundoplication for gastroesophageal reflux disease: a comparative study. BMC Gastroenterol 2020;20(1):162.

31. Yan C, Liang WT, Wang ZG, et al. Comparison of STRETTA procedure and toupet fundoplication for gastroesophageal reflux disease-related extraesophageal symptoms. World J Gastroenterol 2015;21(45):12882–7.

32. Liang WT, Wu JM, Hu ZW, et al. Laparoscopic Nissen fundoplication is more effective in treating patients with GERD-related chronic cough than STRETTA radiofrequency. Minerva Chir 2014;69(3): 121–7.

33. Das B, Reddy M, Khan OA. Is the STRETTA procedure as effective as the best medical and surgical treatments for gastro-oesophageal reflux disease? A best evidence topic. Int J Surg 2016;30:19–24.

34. Ihde GM. The evolution of TIF: transoral incisionless fundoplication. Therap Adv Gastroenterol 2020;13. 1756284820924206.

35. Testoni PA, Testoni S, Distefano G, et al. Transoral incisionless fundoplication with EsophyX for gastroesophageal reflux disease: clinical efficacy is maintained up to 10 years. Endosc Int Open 2019; 7(5):E647–54.

36. Wendling MR, Melvin WS, Perry KA. Impact of transoral incisionless fundoplication (TIF) on subjective and objective GERD indices: a systematic review of the published literature. Surg Endosc 2013; 27(10):3754–61.

37. Hopkins J, Switzer NJ, Karmali S. Update on novel endoscopic therapies to treat gastroesophageal reflux disease: A review. World J Gastrointest Endosc 2015;7(11):1039–44.

38. Richter JE, Kumar A, Lipka S, et al. Efficacy of Laparoscopic Nissen Fundoplication vs Transoral Incisionless Fundoplication or Proton Pump Inhibitors in Patients With Gastroesophageal Reflux Disease: A Systematic Review and Network Meta-analysis. Gastroenterology 2018;154(5):1298–12308 e7.

39. Testoni PA, Testoni S, Mazzoleni G, et al. Long-term efficacy of transoral incisionless fundoplication with Esophyx (Tif 2.0) and factors affecting outcomes in GERD patients followed for up to 6 years: a prospective single-center study. Surg Endosc 2015;29(9): 2770–80.

40. Trad KS, Barnes WE, Simoni G, et al. Transoral incisionless fundoplication effective in eliminating GERD symptoms in partial responders to proton pump inhibitor therapy at 6 months: the TEMPO Randomized Clinical Trial. Surg Innov 2015;22(1): 26–40.

41. Hunter JG, Kahrilas PJ, Bell RC, et al. Efficacy of transoral fundoplication vs omeprazole for treatment of regurgitation in a randomized controlled trial. Gastroenterology 2015;148(2):324–333 e5.

42. Hakansson B, Montgomery M, Cadiere GB, et al. Randomised clinical trial: transoral incisionless fundoplication vs. sham intervention to control chronic GERD. Aliment Pharmacol Ther 2015;42(11–12): 1261–70.

43. Stefanidis G, Viazis N, Kotsikoros N, et al. Long-term benefit of transoral incisionless fundoplication using the esophyx device for the management of gastroesophageal reflux disease responsive to medical therapy. Dis Esophagus 2017;30(3):1–8.

44. Trad KS, Barnes WE, Prevou ER, et al. The TEMPO Trial at 5 Years: Transoral Fundoplication (TIF 2.0) Is Safe, Durable, and Cost-effective. Surg Innov 2018;25(2):149–57.

45. Bell RC, Cadiere GB. Transoral rotational esophagogastric fundoplication: technical, anatomical, and safety considerations. Surg Endosc 2011;25(7): 2387–99.

46. Jain D, Singhal S. Transoral Incisionless Fundoplication for Refractory Gastroesophageal Reflux Disease: Where Do We Stand? Clin Endosc 2016; 49(2):147–56.

# Achalasia
## Surgery Versus Per-Oral Endoscopic Myotomy

Sadia Tasnim, MD[a,b], Siva Raja, MD, PhD[b], Monisha Sudarshan, MD, MPH[b],*

### KEYWORDS

• Achalasia • POEM • Heller myotomy • Dor fundoplication

### KEY POINTS

• Achalasia is a disease with diverse subtypes with type III achalasia forming its own entity.
• Heller myotomy with partial fundoplication has limited outcomes for type III achalasia and per-oral endoscopic myotomy is emerging as the first-line approach.
• Heller myotomy remains the standard operative approach for type II achalasia and in the presence of a diverticulum or hiatal hernia.

## INTRODUCTION

Achalasia is an uncommon esophageal disease characterized by esophageal aperistalsis and incomplete lower esophageal sphincter (LES) relaxation during swallowing. The incidence of achalasia is estimated at 1.6 per 100,000 per year.[1] The cause of achalasia is fairly unknown with one known infectious cause of achalasia being Chagas disease caused by *Trypanosoma cruzi*.[2] The progressive destruction and degeneration of myenteric plexus neurons in the esophagus prevents the LES from relaxing and coordinating peristalsis in different parts of the esophagus. This gives the esophagus a classic "bird's beak" appearance on imaging.

## CLASSIFICATION OF ACHALASIA

Based on manometry, achalasia is classified into 3 types according to the Chicago Classification version 4.0 as shown in **Table 1**.[3,4] Type 1 or classic type is defined as 100% peristalsis without esophageal pressurization. Type 2 (the most common subtype) is defined as pan-esophageal pressurization of more than 30 mm Hg in 20% or more of swallows. Type 3 is defined as premature contractions in 20% or more of swallows with no peristalsis.

Additional categorization of achalasia can be based on morphology (sigmoid vs nonsigmoid[5]) or severity of Eckardt score[6] (**Table 2**).

## OVERVIEW OF MANAGEMENT

Multiple surgical and nonsurgical management options exist for achalasia (**Fig. 1**). Nonsurgical options include pharmacological interventions with nitrates or calcium channel blockers and endoscopic modalities such as pneumatic dilation (PD) and botox injection in the LES.

Botulinum toxin injection can provide significant relief but is temporary, serving a diagnostic and prognostic purpose for other therapies. PD is also effective but short-lived and was the standard treatment of achalasia historically. In our contemporary practice, it is reserved for those who are not surgical candidates. The randomized controlled trial (RCT) by Ponds and colleagues compared 67 patients in the per-oral endoscopic

[a] Digestive Disease and Surgery Institute, Cleveland Clinic Foundation, 9500 Euclid Avenue, Cleveland, OH 44195, USA; [b] Thoracic Surgery, Thoracic and Cardiovascular Surgery Institute, Cleveland Clinic Foundation, 9500 Euclid Avenue, Mail Code J4-1, Cleveland, OH 44195, USA
* Corresponding author.
*E-mail address:* sudarsm2@ccf.org
Twitter: @_SadiaTasnim (S.T.); @Monisha_Sud_MD (M.S.)

Thorac Surg Clin 33 (2023) 135–140
https://doi.org/10.1016/j.thorsurg.2023.01.007
1547-4127/23/© 2023 Elsevier Inc. All rights reserved.

**Table 1**
**Classification of achalasia (Chicago classification version 4.0)**

| Type of Achalasia | Definition |
|---|---|
| Type 1 | Peristalsis without esophageal pressurization or 100% failed peristalsis |
| Type 2 | Pan-esophageal pressurization >30 mm Hg in ≥20% of swallows |
| Type 3 | Premature contractions in ≥20% of swallows with no peristalsis |

*Adapted from* Richter JE. Chicago Classification Version 4.0 and Its Impact on Current Clinical Practice. Gastroenterol Hepatol (N Y). 2021;17(10):468-475.

myotomy (POEM) group and 66 patients in the PD group. An Eckardt score of 3 or less and the absence of severe complications or retreatment at 2-year follow-up was defined as treatment success. This success was noted in 92% of the POEM group but only in 54% of the PD group.[7] Although POEM proved to be significantly more effective in this trial, the trial used a 30 to 35 mm not a 40-mm balloon, which has been demonstrated to have up to an 86% success at 2 years in other studies.[8]

Surgical options for achalasia include POEM and Heller myotomy. Thoracoscopic Heller myotomy was first introduced in the United States by Pelligrini in 1991 and later evolved to incorporate an antireflux element or fundoplication.[9] POEM was first described in Japan in 2010 and continues to grow for a selected patient population.[5] Although a Heller myotomy has served as the front-line surgical approach in achalasia, we know that with such a diverse disease spectrum, there is no standard approach.

## OUR APPROACH TO PER-ORAL ENDOSCOPIC MYOTOMY AND HELLER MYOTOMY WITH DOR FUNDOPLICATION
### Heller Myotomy with Fundoplication

We prefer a supine split leg position with a midline periumbilical port placed for the camera. Four additional ports are placed in the hypochondrium, first for liver retraction, second and third are working ports, and the fourth is the assistant port. The gastro-hepatic ligament is divided using thermal coagulation. We tend to limit circumferential gastroesophageal junction (GEJ) dissection and focus on the anterior part if there is no significant hiatal hernia component. The trajectory of the vagus nerve is followed and preserved at all times.

The GEJ fat pad is removed. There are several methods to perform a safe myotomy. Our approach is primarily robotic (**Fig. 2**) and thus we use gentle separation of the muscle fibers using a grasper and low cautery as our preferred method. At all times, energy is kept away from the esophageal mucosa to prevent a full thickness injury. A complete myotomy of the longitudinal and circular muscle fibers is performed. Dissection is carried 6 to 8 cm proximally and 3 to 4 cm distally from the GEJ. Intraoperative endoscopy can be used to check for leaks and to ensure that sufficient myotomy has been performed by assessing the relaxation of the GEJ. Partial fundoplication is performed after Heller myotomy (see **Fig. 2**A) with our preference being a 3-stitch Dor fundoplication (see **Fig. 2**B). Patients are started on clear liquids the day after surgery following a gastrografin swallow test and are dismissed home shortly thereafter.

### Per-Oral Endoscopic Myotomy

We usually perform an anterior myotomy unless the patient underwent a prior Heller procedure in which case a posterior myotomy is performed. We have previously described our approach to POEM as shown in **Fig. 3**.[6,10]

A submucosal tunnel is created starting approximately 10 to 12 cm proximal to the LES and extending to about 2 to 4 cm into the gastric side. Myotomy of the circular muscle fibers is started 2 to 4 cm distally from the mucosotomy to create a flap. The myotomy is extended 2 to 4 cm into the gastric wall. Mucosotomy closure is performed tightly with endoscopic clips. On postoperative day 1, an esophagram is performed to rule out transmural perforations. If no complications are found, patients are started on a clear liquid diet, twice daily proton pump inhibitor for 2 months, and are advised to advance the diet gradually during the next 1 to 2 weeks.

## PER-ORAL ENDOSCOPIC MYOTOMY VERSUS HELLER MYOTOMY WITH FUNDOPLICATION

Our understanding of achalasia has deepened during the past few decades because we realize the disease lies over a spectrum with significant variability over each subtype. Type III achalasia may be considered an entity by itself, distinguishing itself from other subtypes. We are also aware that achalasia is a progressive disease that worsens with or without intervention. For these reasons, there is no singular solution for achalasia, and intervention needs to be customized.

The debate between POEM and Heller myotomy is misplaced because the question is not which

**Table 2**
**Eckardt scale**

| Score | Weight Loss (kg) | Dysphagia | Retrosternal Pain | Regurgitation |
|-------|------------------|-----------|-------------------|---------------|
| 0 | None | None | None | None |
| 1 | <5 | Occasional | Occasional | Occasional |
| 2 | 5–10 | Daily | Daily | Daily |
| 3 | >10 | Each meal | Each meal | Each meal |

intervention is better suitable for achalasia but rather when. **Fig. 4** depicts an algorithm to help guide such a decision.

There are several studies that have reported the limited benefit of Heller myotomy for type III achalasia. Symptom recurrence after Heller myotomy is higher at 30% for type III achalasia compared with only 4.6% for type II achalasia.[11] Patients with type II achalasia have a nearly 4.6 times increase in treatment success after Heller in comparison with type III achalasia. The limited palliative effect of traditional therapies for type III achalasia is possibly attributed to the shorter myotomy being performed, which has pushed POEM to the forefront for this subtype.

We have previously published our outcomes for POEM in type III achalasia, which is our first-line choice of treatment of this subtype. POEM provides a longer myotomy to address the lumen obliterating midesophageal spasms of type III achalasia. In our retrospective review of POEM used for type III achalasia in 35 patients, we found a significant decrease in Eckhart scores and improvements in LES pressures, 1-minute barium column height, and 1-minute barium column width.[12]

We also elect to use POEM for patients with type I achalasia because there is a concern that fundoplication decreases the effectiveness of the myotomy given the amotility of the esophagus. However, a severely sigmoidal or sink trap esophagus prevents optimal visualization for an endoscopic myotomy, and in these cases, we opt for a Heller myotomy without fundoplication. In addition, patients with hiatal hernia or a significant epiphrenic diverticulum receive a Heller myotomy in order to complete the adjunct procedures associated with these conditions. Our current institutional data (publication pending) suggest POEM and Heller myotomy provide comparable short-term outcomes for selected patients with type I achalasia.

Werner and colleagues completed a multicenter RCT of POEM versus surgical Heller myotomy with Dor fundoplication with 221 patients during a 2-year follow-up period.[13] Clinical success was

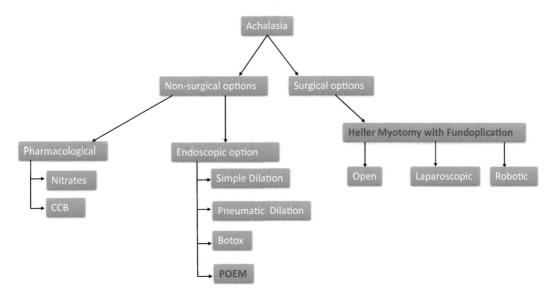

**Fig. 1.** Achalasia treatment options.

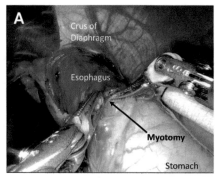
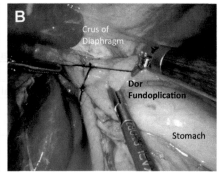

**Fig. 2.** Heller myotomy (*A*) and Dor fundoplication (*B*).

defined as an Eckhardt score of less than 3 with success in 83% of the POEM group and 81.7% in the surgical myotomy group thus demonstrating noninferiority of POEM. The prevalence of type III was only 8% to 11% within the cohorts, and as discussed earlier, this subtype has limited outcomes with Heller myotomy. Reflux esophagitis was present in 44% of the POEM cohort and 29% in the surgical myotomy group seen on endoscopy at 2 years. Certainly, the prevalence of reflux esophagitis is higher in POEM, and once again, the long-term implications of this finding remain to be elucidated. In our current experience, most patients with reflux are well-controlled with medication, and the need to perform a fundoplication has been rare.

POEM also remains an excellent rescue option for symptom recurrence after a previous myotomy offering a virgin plane for the redo myotomy. For Heller myotomy recurrences, our preference is to perform a posterior myotomy thus avoiding the previous dissection plane and the wrap.

In general, patients that are not suitable surgical candidates due to advanced age, comorbidities, and frozen abdomen secondary to previous surgeries are offered POEM over Heller myotomy.

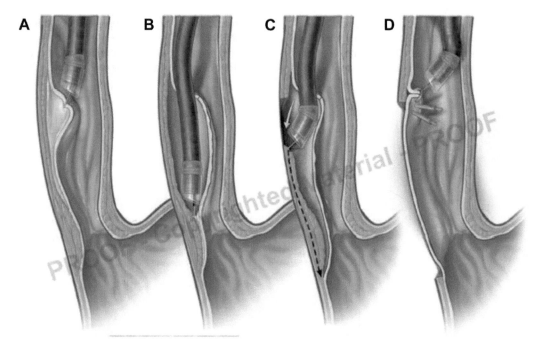

**Fig. 3.** Steps of POEM. (*A*) Mucosal incision and injection of 10 cc of indigo carmine strained normal saline in the submucosa, (*B*) Creating of submucosal tunnel, (*C*) inner circular muscle sometimes of the longitudinal muscle myotomy, and (*D*) mucosotomy closure with endoclips. (Reprinted with permission, Cleveland Clinic Foundation ©2020. All Rights Reserved.)

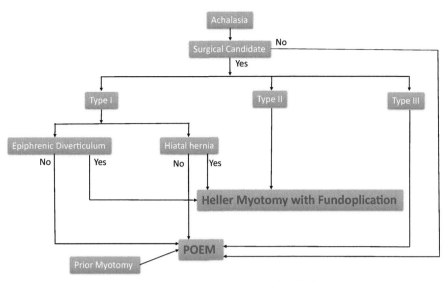

**Fig. 4.** Decision flow chart POEM versus Heller myotomy with Dor fundoplication.

## SUMMARY

Achalasia is a disease with a wide spectrum and distinct subtypes with type III forming its own entity. The time-dependent failure of achalasia adds to the complexity of the disease. Due to these issues, there is no singular palliation for achalasia with each case requiring a custom approach. The 2 most central palliative treatments are Heller myotomy and POEM. We find a POEM is most suitable for type III achalasia, salvage myotomy, and select type I achalasia. We reserve Heller myotomy via a minimally invasive approach for type II achalasia, presence of a hiatal hernia, epiphrenic diverticulum, or a sink trap esophagus. Currently, rates of reflux esophagitis are up to 50% after POEM with operative fundoplication rarely necessary. As 5 to 10-year data become available, longer-term outcomes of achalasia and different palliative approaches will be revealed.

## CLINICS CARE POINTS

- A customized approach to palliation of achalasia is key in optimizing outcomes.
- The POEM procedure is better suited for type III achalasia due to a longer myotomy, providing effective palliation of lumen obliterating spasms.
- Type II achalasia, presence of an epiphrenic diverticulum or hiatal hernia is better managed with a Heller myotomy with fundoplication.

## DISCLOSURES

The authors have nothing to disclose.

## REFERENCES

1. Sadowski DC, Ackah F, Jiang B, et al. Achalasia: incidence, prevalence and survival. A population-based study. Neurogastroenterol Motil 2010;22(9): e256–61.
2. Martins RK, Ribeiro IB, De Moura DTH, et al. Peroral (poem) or surgical myotomy for the treatment of achalasia: a systematic review and meta-analysis. Arq Gastroenterol 2020;57(1):79–86. Available at: https://pubmed.ncbi.nlm.nih.gov/32294740/. Accessed July 20, 2022.
3. Khan A, Yadlapati R, Gonlachanvit S, et al. Chicago Classification update (version 4.0): technical review on diagnostic criteria for achalasia. Neuro Gastroenterol Motil 2021;33(7):e14182.
4. Richter JE. Chicago classification version 4.0 and its impact on current clinical practice. Gastroenterol Hepatol 2021;17(10):468–75.
5. Inoue H, Minami H, Kobayashi Y, et al. Peroral endoscopic myotomy (POEM) for esophageal achalasia. Endoscopy 2010;42(4):265–71.
6. Sanaka MR, Jegadeesan R, Thota PN, et al. Two-person technique of peroral endoscopic myotomy for achalasia with an advanced endoscopist and a thoracic surgeon: initial experience. Can J Gastroenterol Hepatol 2016;2016:1–6.
7. Ponds FA, Fockens P, Lei A, et al. Effect of peroral endoscopic myotomy vs pneumatic dilation on symptom severity and treatment outcomes among treatment-naive patients with achalasia: a randomized clinical trial. JAMA 2019;322(2):134–44.

8. Moonen A, Annese V, Belmans A, et al. Long-term results of the European achalasia trial: a multicentre randomised controlled trial comparing pneumatic dilation versus laparoscopic Heller myotomy. Gut 2016;65(5):732–9.
9. Patti MG, Andolfi C, Bowers SP, et al. POEM vs Laparoscopic heller myotomy and fundoplication: which is now the gold standard for treatment of achalasia? J Gastrointest Surg 2017;21(2):207–14.
10. Chadalavada P, Thota PN, Raja S, et al. Peroral endoscopic myotomy as a novel treatment for achalasia: patient selection and perspectives. Clin Exp Gastroenterol 2020;13:485–95.
11. Salvador R, Costantini M, Zaninotto G, et al. The preoperative manometric pattern predicts the outcome of surgical treatment for esophageal achalasia. J Gastrointest Surg 2010;14(11):1635–45.
12. Sudarshan M, Raja S, Adhikari S, et al. Peroral endoscopic myotomy provides effective palliation in type III achalasia. J Thorac Cardiovasc Surg 2022; 163(2):512–9.e1.
13. Werner YB, Hakanson B, Martinek J, et al. Endoscopic or surgical myotomy in patients with idiopathic achalasia. N Engl J Med 2019;381(23): 2219–29.

# Tracheobronchoplasty
## Indications and Best Approaches

Richard Lazzaro, MD[a],*, Matthew L. Inra, MD[b]

## KEYWORDS

- Tracheobronchomalacia • Robotic tracheobronchoplasty • Excessive central airway collapse
- Pulmonary function test

## KEY POINTS

- Tracheobronchomalacia (TBM) is an increasingly recognized abnormality of the central airways. Patients with persistent respiratory symptoms despite optimal medical therapy should be screened for TBM.
- Dynamic computerized tomography (CT) protocols with ultralow-dose forced exhalation imaging with cinematic reconstructions are a valuable screening tool for patients with suspected TBM.
- Awake dynamic bronchoscopy remains the gold standard to diagnose TBM.
- Robotic-assisted minimally invasive tracheobronchoplasty is safe, improves function, improves quality of life, and is less morbid than the open approach with the goal of surgery being to restore the C-shaped configuration of the airway and pleating the lax posterior membrane to the mesh for objective and subjective symptomatic improvement.

 Video content accompanies this article at http://www.thoracic.theclinics.com.

## INTRODUCTION/BACKGROUND/PREVALENCE

Excessive central airway collapse (ECAC) comprises 2 distinct morphologic entities that can be readily identified and assessed for its contribution to an individual's symptoms of cough, recurrent infection, or shortness of breath. During exhalation, the cross-sectional area of the central airways (trachea, main bronchi and bronchus intermedius) will radially contract as the intrathoracic pressure is elevated resulting in increased transtracheal pressure and airway narrowing. A reduction in tracheal diameter of greater than 50% during exhalation is considered abnormal.[1–3] During normal or forced exhalation in patients with ECAC, the elevated transtracheal pressure results in abnormal degrees of airway collapse.[4] ECAC has different severities; it is defined as mild if there is 70% to 80% collapse of the luminal cross-sectional area, moderate if there is 81% to 90%

collapse and severe if there is greater than 90% collapse.[5,6] ECAC includes a spectrum of disease manifestations that include tracheobronchomalacia (TBM) and excessive dynamic airway collapse (EDAC).

"TBM is an increasingly recognized abnormality of the central airways in patients with respiratory complaints."[5] The cause of TBM is multifactorial, involving patient and environmental factors. An association of TBM with the utilization of inhaled corticosteroids in higher doses and prolonged duration has been reported.[7] TBM is characterized by changes in the shape of the central trachea and/or bronchi. The normal C-shape of the trachea and bronchi seen on cross-sectional imaging or bronchoscopy is replaced by narrowing to the anteroposterior dimension of the trachea and/or bronchi with simultaneous widening of the lateral dimension or width of the airway. This change in shape results in a crescent-shaped trachea often

[a] Thoracic Surgery, Southern Region Robert Wood Johnson Barnabas Health, 1 Robert Wood Johnson Pl, New Brunswick, NJ 08901, USA; [b] 130 East 77th Street, 4th Floor, New York, NY 10075, USA
* Corresponding author. 67 Route 37 West Toms River, NJ 08755.
*E-mail address:* rlazzaro@mac.com

Thorac Surg Clin 33 (2023) 141–147
https://doi.org/10.1016/j.thorsurg.2023.01.001
1547-4127/23/© 2023 Elsevier Inc. All rights reserved.

referred to as a "frown" with either tidal breathing or forced exhalation. More importantly, this change in shape results in a reduction of the cross-sectional area of the airway.[1,5,8] EDAC is characterized by the preservation of the C-shaped trachea and bronchi. During tidal or forced exhalation, the cartilaginous structure is preserved; atrophy of the posterior membrane, composed of the trachealis muscle, results in an excessive anterior displacement of the posterior membrane, which again decreases the cross-sectional area of the central airways. For the purposes of this discussion, we will focus the discussion on TBM in adults.

The prevalence of TBM in an adult is difficult to quantify.[9] TBM is infrequently considered as a clinical condition or a condition contributing to a patient's symptoms of cough, recurrent infection, or shortness of breath. The symptoms of cough, bronchitis, and shortness of breath, which are the primary symptoms of TBM, are often attributed to more common pulmonary diseases such as chronic obstructive pulmonary disease (COPD) and asthma. Although TBM causes many of the same symptoms as is seen in COPD and asthma, there is neither a specific pattern of pulmonary function test (PFT) results nor a diagnostic criterion on pulmonary function testing for patients with TBM.[10] PFTs in patients with TBM can show "diminished expiratory flow, typical notching on the flow-volume (FV) loop, dynamic airway compression (calculated as slow vital capacity minus forced vital capacity [FVC]), a biphasic FV loop or flow oscillations (and) these findings are neither sensitive nor specific."[1] Often, patients with TBM have normal FV loops, and PFT's should not be used to diagnose or determine the severity of disease in patients diagnosed with TBM.[10,11]

TBM is important to diagnose because it is a treatable condition but it may well be underdiagnosed in the current population of patients presenting with its typical symptoms. COPD, which is present in many of these patients, seems to provide sufficient reason for respiratory distress and the typical symptoms.[4] TBM coexist in patients with COPD and other obstructive airway diseases. A retrospective review of patients with COPD showed a prevalence of TBM in 8.4% of patients with COPD and 9.2% of patients with asthma on their inspiratory CT scans.[12] Although it is possible to diagnose TBM on inspiratory imaging, the identification of TBM using routine (breath hold) CT imaging is not adequate in screening for the disease and, as a result, may decrease the true prevalence of TBM if the clinician ordering the test does not have an increased index of suspicion for the diagnosis. Additional expiratory imaging will demonstrate additional cases of central airway collapse.

Sverzellati and colleagues identified airway malacia in 53% of patients with stable COPD undergoing end inspiratory and dynamic expiratory imaging.[13] The prevalence of COPD, among people aged 30 to 79 years is as high as 10.3%,[14] and there is an association or coexistence of TBM with COPD and other obstructive airway diseases, so TBM must be considered to be more prevalent than currently identified in the population. It should be considered in the differential diagnosis for patients with progressive or intractable symptoms of cough, dyspnea with exertion, or recurrent pneumonia, whether the patients already carry a diagnosis of COPD or asthma.

### Patient Evaluation Overview

Patients with persistent or progressive symptoms of cough, recurrent infections, and shortness of breath, after optimization of current diagnoses such as COPD and asthma, need a workup for central airway disease. This workup includes a dynamic CT scan and/or awake dynamic bronchoscopy. Dynamic CT images are best acquired with a multidetector helical CT scanner during forceful exhalation. The technologist should coach the patient during the exhalation phase as images are acquired. Inspiratory and expiratory images are measured to compare the central airway cross-sectional area during each phase. Ultralow-dose dynamic protocols have been developed to limit radiation exposure without compromise of image quality.[15] Cross-sectional area of the trachea and central bronchi are measured during inhalation and forced exhalation. The measurements are compared, and the percent dynamic collapse is calculated. Cinematic reconstructions are additive and provide a visual representation of the dynamic collapse (Video 1).

Awake dynamic bronchoscopy is considered the gold standard to confirm the diagnosis, severity, and extent of TBM.[9,16,17] It is performed under light sedation with topical anesthesia to eliminate gag reflex and cough because this may overestimate the amount of narrowing. This test provides real-time visualization of the airways and narrowing, and dynamic CT imaging has been shown to be concordant with dynamic bronchoscopy in up to 97% of patients.[18]

Short-term airway stenting with silicone[1,19] and metallic stents[20] has been performed to assess for symptom improvement and/or resolution of symptoms with the goal of improving patient selection for definitive surgical repair, or tracheobronchoplasty (TBP).[21] Short-term stenting is not an ideal diagnostic test as stents can migrate, obstruct, and cause symptoms[10,22]; additionally, short-term stenting may not provide a long enough trial period to predict amelioration of symptoms following stent explantation and definitive surgical repair, TBP. The authors infrequently use temporary stenting as diagnosis and surgical candidacy can be determined without it but when used, it should be used selectively for the reasons discussed earlier.

After evaluation and diagnosis as described earlier, TBP is recommended to symptomatic patients with severe TBM (**Fig. 1**).

## History of Tracheobronchoplasty

In 1954, Nissen and Herzog described tightening the posterior membranous wall and reinforcing the repair with bone grafts.[23] The modern revision of this technique uses permanent mesh along the membranous wall acting as a posterior splint. This mesh allows in-growth of tissue without erosion into neighboring structures.[4,6,21] Historically, a high right posterolateral thoracotomy provided the necessary exposure of the intrathoracic trachea and bilateral bronchi. The morbidity associated with the open approach limited the application of TBP to very few patients, and the performance to fewer surgeons and institutions.

As surgery has evolved to embrace minimally invasive techniques, so has TBP. In 2011, Tse and colleagues described their video-assisted TBP for TBM, repairing the trachea and right-sided bronchus and placed uncovered metallic stents in the left main bronchus in 2 patients.[24] In 2013, the author (RL) performed the first robotic-assisted minimally invasive bilateral bronchoplasty for severe TBM.[9] In 2016, the author (RL) published the experience of robotic-assisted TBP for 42 patients with severe symptomatic TBM; this series was the first of its kind in the world.[6]

## Operative Technique

The goal of surgical repair is to restore the C-shaped configuration of the airway lumen and splint or secure the lax posterior membrane to the mesh. Perioperative antibiotics are administered, and sterile technique is used throughout the procedure. The patient is induced under general anesthesia and intubated with a 35 French (Fr) double lumen endotracheal tube to selectively ventilate the left lung. The patient is placed in the left lateral decubitus position. We use preemptive analgesia at the incision sites and perform multiple intercostal nerve blocks under direct visualization following the initial access. We use a 4-arm robotic approach with a fifth port for the assistant (**Fig. 2**, Video 2). The pleural space is insufflated with carbon dioxide ($CO_2$) at a pressure of 8 mm Hg and a flow of 8 L/min. The procedure is divided into 3 distinct stages. Stage I involves division of tissue anterior to the esophagus with careful application of cautery from the level of the inferior pulmonary

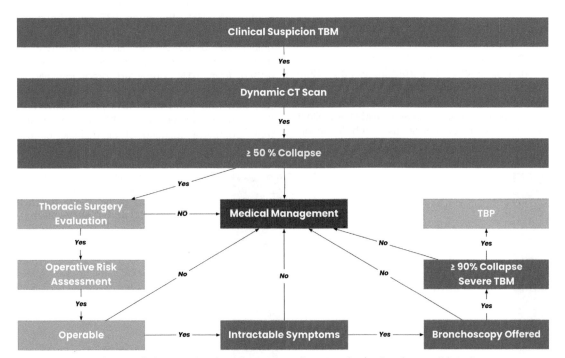

**Fig. 1.** Patient evaluation following the clinical suspicion of TBM and selection for candidacy for TBP.

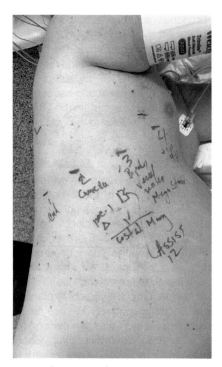

**Fig. 2.** Port placement. The assistant, 12-mm port, is positioned at the inferior vertex of an isosceles triangle drawn from the second and third robotic ports to the costal margin. The assistant port is positioned under direct visualization in a supradiaphragmatic position and is used for suture passing as well as mesh. Instrumentation for robotic repair and the associated ports is shown.

ligament to the thoracic inlet, dividing the azygous vein. Meticulous hemostasis is beneficial because this optimizes visualization. Stage II involves subcarinal lymphadenectomy from the left mainstem bronchus to the carina, and then along the right mainstem bronchus and bronchus intermedius. Removing this nodal packet provides excellent visualization of the central airways. With $CO_2$ insuf-

flation, the mediastinum is displaced leftward and with the fourth arm of the robot, gentle traction is applied to retract the right lung anteriorly, bringing the entirety of the left mainstem bronchus in view (**Fig. 3**). Stage III involves the performance of the posterior splinting TBP. A prolene mesh, cut to a 5-cm length and 16-mm width, is secured to the left main bronchus with 3 columns of 4 to 0 vicryl suture on an RB-1 needle. Performing the left mainstem bronchus repair requires communication between the surgeon and the anesthesiologist because intermittent apnea and repositioning of the endotracheal tube under surgeon guidance is used until the left bronchoplasty is completed. The tracheal prolene mesh is often 8 cm in length by 24 mm in width and is secured to the trachea with 4 columns of 4 to 0 vicryl sutures on an RB-1 needle. Finally, the right mainstem bronchus and bronchus intermedius are repaired with a prolene mesh the same size as the left mainstem mesh and 4 to 0 vicryl sutures on an RB-1 needle are used (**Figs. 4 and 5**). Following repair, a 24 (Fr) chest tube is inserted, and the patient is extubated in the supine position under bronchoscopic visualization to assess the repair. A detailed description of the robotic technique has been described.[25]

## FUNCTIONAL AND QUALITY OF LIFE OUTCOMES IN OPEN TRACHEOBRONCHOMALACIA SURGERY

Both changes in PFTs and quality of life for patients with TBM after open TBP have been reported. Following open TBP, Wright and colleagues demonstrated an improvement in mean forced expiratory volume in 1 second (FEV1) from 51% predicted preoperatively to 73% postoperatively ($P = .009$), and peak expiratory flow rate (PEF) from 49% preoperatively to 70% postoperatively ($P < .00001$), concluding that "complete splinting of all malacic central

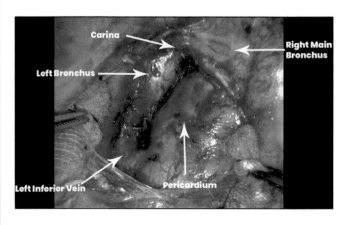

**Fig. 3.** Following Esophageal Mobilization, and lymphadenectomy, the left main bronchus, carina, distal trachea and right main bronchus are visualized.

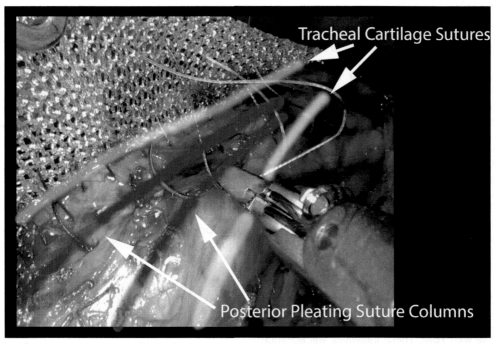

**Fig. 4.** The tracheal membranous pleating sutures are shown in a partial thickness placement through the trachealis muscle.

airways with Marlex restores anatomic configuration and permanently prevents expiratory collapse, with relief of extreme dyspnea, cough, and secretion retention."[4] Significant improvement in St George Respiratory Questionnaire scores, dyspnea indexes, Karnofsky performance status, and 6-minute walk duration have been reported following open TBP as well.[26]

## OUTCOMES OF ROBOTIC TRACHEOBRONCHOPLASTY

Subsequent report of the first series of 42 patients undergoing robotic tracheobronchoplasty (R-TBP) demonstrated safety of the robotic repair and

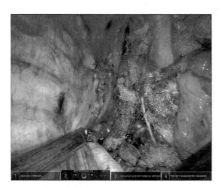

**Fig. 5.** Completed TBP.

short-term efficacy. There was no 90-day mortality. There were a total of 19 postoperative complications within the first 90 days, including 11 minor complications (26%) and 8 major complications (19%) as defined by Clavien-Dindo classification schema.[6] All patients were discharged to home, and the need for postoperative bronchoscopy for tracheobronchial hygiene was 2.4%. Median hospital length of stay was 3 days. At a median follow-up of 4 months, FEV1 increased by 13.5% (P = .01), FVC increased by 14.5% (P < .0001), and PEF increased by 21.0% (P < .0001). Patient quality of life was improved postoperatively when compared with preoperative baseline.[6] Results of the intermediate follow-up of this initial cohort of 42 patients at a median follow-up of 29 months revealed that sustained improvements in FEV1 (preoperative median: 74% vs postoperative median: 82%, P = .001), FVC (preoperative median: 68.5% vs postoperative median: 80.63%, P < .001), and PEF (preoperative median: 61.5% vs postoperative median: 75%, P = .02).[27] In addition, there was a significant decrease in SGRQ total score (preoperative median: 65.28 vs postoperative median: 34. P = .001), SGRQ symptom score (preoperative median: 82.6 vs postoperative median: 43.99 P < .001), and SQRQ impact score (preoperative median: 55.78 vs postoperative median: 25.95 P < .001).[27]

## SUMMARY

TBM is a hugely underdiagnosed disease. Often patients with COPD and asthma are treated for their respiratory symptoms with escalations in therapy while consideration for ECAC has not been explored. Dynamic CT scan protocols provide a screening test central airway collapse in patients with cough, recurrent pulmonary infections, and shortness of breath. Awake dynamic bronchoscopy remains the gold standard to diagnose ECAC, and should be used for the patient with progressive symptoms refractory to current medical treatments. The robotic-assisted minimally invasive TBP is the ideal approach to definitively repair the central airways for patients with severe symptomatic TBM because it is safe and improves PFTs and patient quality of life with durability of results at intermediate follow-up.

A multi-institutional TBM patient registry and multidisciplinary TBM expertise group of pulmonologists, radiologists, interventional pulmonologists, and thoracic surgeons will be invaluable to patients with TBM. These initiatives will advance physician knowledge of TBM as a disease through collaborative investigation and research. These advances include, but are not limited to, improving diagnosis in at risk patient populations and finally standardizing a treatment approach, including timing of TBP.

## CLINICS CARE POINTS

- TBM is an increasingly recognized abnormality of the central airways
- Dynamic CT protocols with ultralow-dose forced exhalation imaging are used to screen patients with suspected TBM, using cinematic reconstructions
- Awake dynamic bronchoscopy is still the gold standard to diagnose TBM
- Robotic-assisted minimally invasive TBP is safe, improves function, improves quality of life, and is less morbid than the open approach
- The goal of surgery is to restore the C-shaped configuration of the airway and splint or secure the lax posterior membrane to the mesh
- The operative procedure has 3 distinct stages
  - Stage I Exposure of the airway through anterior dissection of the esophagus from the inferior pulmonary ligament to the thoracic inlet
  - Stage II Subcarinal lymph node dissection to expose the carina and bilateral bronchi
  - Stage III Airway repair utilizing mesh
- Development of a multidisciplinary TBM expertise group
- Development of a multi-institutional TBM patient registry

## DECLARATION OF INTERESTS

No relevant disclosures.

## SUPPLEMENTARY DATA

Supplementary data related to this article can be found online at https://doi.org/10.1016/j.thorsurg.2023.01.001.

## REFERENCES

1. Murgu SD, Colt HG. Tracheobronchomalacia and excessive dynamic airway collapse. Respirology 2006;11(4):388–406.
2. Campbell AH, Faulks LW. Expiratory air-flow pattern in tracheobronchial collapse. Am Rev Respir Dis 1965;92(5):781–91.
3. Johnson TH, Mikita JJ, Wilson JJ, et al. Acquired tracheomalacia. Radiology 1973;109(3):576–80.
4. Wright CD, Grillo HC, Hammoud T, et al. Tracheoplasty for expiratory collapse of central airways. Ann Thorac Surg 2005;80(1):259–66.
5. Buitrago DH, Wilson JL, Parikh A, et al. Current concepts in severe adult tracheobronchomalacia: evaluation and treatment. J Thorac Dis 2017;9(1):E57–66.
6. Lazzaro R, Patton B, Lee P, et al. First series of minimally invasive, robot-assisted tracheobronchoplasty with mesh for severe tracheobronchomalacia. J Thorac Cardiovasc Surg 2019;157(2):791–800.
7. Shah V, Husta B, Mehta A, et al. Association between inhaled corticosteroids and tracheobronchomalacia. Chest 2020.
8. Murgu S, Colt H. Tracheobronchomalacia and excessive dynamic airway collapse. Clin Chest Med 2013;34(3):527–55.
9. Lazar JF, Posner DH, Palka W, et al. Robotically assisted bilateral bronchoplasty for tracheobronchomalacia. Innovations (Phila) 2015;10(6):428–30.
10. Wright CD. Tracheobronchomalacia and expiratory collapse of central airways. Thorac Surg Clin 2018;28(2):163–6.
11. Majid A, Sosa AF, Ernst A, et al. Pulmonary function and flow-volume loop patterns in patients with tracheobronchomalacia. Respir Care 2013;58(9):1521–6.
12. Patel RIL, Patel V, Esan A, et al. The prevalence of tracheobronchomalacia in patients with asthma or

chronic obstructive pulmonary disease. Internet J Pulm Med 2010;12(1):1–5.

13. Sverzellati N, Rastelli A, Chetta A, et al. Airway malacia in chronic obstructive pulmonary disease: prevalence, morphology and relationship with emphysema, bronchiectasis and bronchial wall thickening. Eur Radiol 2009;19(7):1669–78.

14. Adeloye D, Song P, Zhu Y, et al. Global, regional, and national prevalence of, and risk factors for, chronic obstructive pulmonary disease (COPD) in 2019: a systematic review and modelling analysis. Lancet Respir Med 2022;10(5):447–58.

15. Cohen SL, Ben-Levi E, Karp JB, et al. Ultralow dose dynamic expiratory computed tomography for evaluation of tracheomalacia. J Comput Assist Tomogr 2019;43(2):307–11.

16. Abia-Trujillo D, Majid A, Johnson M, et al. Central airway collapse, an underappreciated cause of respiratory morbidity. Mayo Clin Proc 2020;95(12): 2747–54.

17. Kheir F, Majid A. Tracheobronchomalacia and excessive dynamic airway collapse: medical and surgical treatment. Semin Respir Crit Care Med 2018;39(6):667–73.

18. Lee KS, Sun MRM, Ernst A, et al. Comparison of dynamic expiratory CT with bronchoscopy for diagnosing airway malacia: a pilot evaluation. Chest 2007;131(3):758–64.

19. Ernst A, Majid A, Feller-Kopman D, et al. Airway stabilization with silicone stents for treating adult tracheobronchomalacia: a prospective observational study. Chest 2007;132(2):609–16.

20. Majid A, Alape D, Kheir F, et al. Short-term use of uncovered self-expanding metallic airway stents for severe expiratory central airway collapse. Respiration 2016;92(6):389–96.

21. Gangadharan SP, Bakhos CT, Majid A, et al. Technical aspects and outcomes of tracheobronchoplasty for severe tracheobronchomalacia. Ann Thorac Surg 2011;91(5):1574–80 [discussion: 1580–1].

22. Wright CD, Mathisen DJ. Tracheobronchoplasty for tracheomalacia. Ann Cardiothorac Surg 2018;7(2): 261–5.

23. Herzog HNR. Relaxation an expiratory invagination of the membranous portion of the intrathoracic trachea and the main bronchi as a cause of asphyxia attacks in bronchial asthma and the chronic asthmoid bronchitis of pulmonary emphysema. Schweiz Med Wochenschr 1954;(84):217–21.

24. Tse DG, Han SM, Charuworn B, et al. Video-assisted thoracoscopic surgical tracheobronchoplasty for tracheobronchomalacia. J Thorac Cardiovasc Surg 2011;142(3):714–6.

25. Lazzaro RS, Bahrloomi D, Wasserman GA, et al. Robotic tracheobronchoplasty: technique. Oper Tech Thorac Cardiovasc Surg 2022;27(2):218–26.

26. Gangadharan SP. Tracheobronchomalacia in adults. Semin Thorac Cardiovasc Surg 2010;22(2):165–73.

27. Lazzaro RS, Patton BD, Wasserman GA, et al. Robotic-assisted tracheobronchoplasty: quality of life and pulmonary function assessment on intermediate follow-up. J Thorac Cardiovasc Surg 2022;164(1): 278–86.

# Pulmonary Metastasectomy
## Indications, Best Practices, and Evolving Role in the Future

Michael Eisenberg, MD, Nathaniel Deboever, MD, Mara B. Antonoff, MD*

## KEYWORDS

• Pulmonary metastases • Metastasectomy • Lung resection

## KEY POINTS

- Pulmonary metastasectomy affords appropriately selected patients the opportunity for local control, resulting in freedom from systemic therapy, prolonged disease-free intervals, and even cure from disease and improved overall survival.
- In general, pulmonary metastasectomy tends to be most beneficial when primary tumors are fully eradicated, all pulmonary metastatic disease can be controlled locally, and there is no evidence of active extrathoracic metastases.
- As compared with surgical resection for non–small cell lung cancer, parenchymal-sparing techniques should be emphasized.

## INTRODUCTION/HISTORY/DEFINITIONS/BACKGROUND

For patients with extrapulmonary primary malignancies, the lung is the most frequent site of metastatic spread.[1] Pulmonary metastatic disease occurs frequently in colorectal cancer (CRC), sarcoma, melanoma, head and neck cancers, breast cancer, and tumors of the urinary tract, with numerous other malignancies known to additionally spread to the lungs.[2,3] Historically, systemic therapy has been considered standard of care for stage IV cancer, given the systemic nature of the disease; however, options for local therapy for metastatic pulmonary nodules are expanding, with substantial evidence for efficacy in terms of optimal local control for prolonging life, delaying recurrence, and enabling patients to experience freedom from chemotherapy.[4]

With regard to the benefits of local therapy for pulmonary metastatic disease, the existing literature is challenging to interpret, given the broad heterogeneity of the populations included, spanning numerous histologies, extents of disease burden, and types of treatment.[5] Even within focused series, there are vast differences among patient outcomes related to the type of surgical resection or modality of ablative therapy.[2,4,6,7] Although it may be inappropriate to offer local therapy to all patients with pulmonary metastatic disease, it is well established that there are substantial benefits that local therapy may provide to a highly selected subgroup of patients. Evaluation of candidacy is best addressed in a multidisciplinary fashion, with input from the full care team. More specifically, in addressing the role of surgery for pulmonary metastatic disease, there are several highly relevant questions that must be considered: (1) Is this disease biology appropriate for local therapy? (2) Is this patient a good physiologic and anatomic candidate for surgery? (3) What is the optimal timing for providing local therapy to this patient? (4) Is surgery the most suitable local modality for treating this patient?

Department of Thoracic and Cardiovascular Surgery, University of Texas MD Anderson Cancer Center, 1515 Holcombe Boulevard, Houston, TX 77030, USA
* Corresponding author.
*E-mail address:* mbantonoff@MDAnderson.org

Thorac Surg Clin 33 (2023) 149–158
https://doi.org/10.1016/j.thorsurg.2023.01.004
1547-4127/23/© 2023 Elsevier Inc. All rights reserved.

Pertaining to disease biology, it is known that certain tumor histologies tend to lead to prolonged disease-free intervals (DFIs) after local therapy, whereas others tend to recur quickly. In general, the demonstration of disease stability and absence of extrathoracic metastases are well accepted as factors that are associated with better outcomes after local therapy.[8] Furthermore, the ability to locally address all sites of disease is a particularly important consideration with regard to higher-risk interventions.[1] Although there is no upper limit on number of pulmonary metastases that may be resected, it has been demonstrated (eg, in CRC) that the presence of greater than three pulmonary nodules at the first metastasectomy increases likelihood of subsequent pulmonary recurrence.[9] Nonetheless, resections of greater numbers of lesions have been safely performed with favorable outcomes, and the total number is less relevant than the ability to perform an R0 resection with an extent of lung removed that is tolerated by the individual patient. Finally, it is relevant to consider that some tumors have alternative management strategies that are well tolerated by patients, such as those who can be managed by oral hormonal agents, whereas other diseases may be treatable only by highly toxic chemotherapeutic agents or may not even be treatable with systemic drugs at all. All these elements of disease biology are pertinent to the discussion of offering local therapy.

As with therapeutic interventions for any medical condition, one must consider not only the best way to treat the disease but also whether the patient is an appropriate candidate for the treatment. For pulmonary resection, patient comorbidities are particularly germane, because this may often weigh heavily in the decision as to which form of local therapy is offered. For patients to be surgical candidates, one must consider pulmonary reserve, frailty, and general ability to tolerate a general anesthetic and the surgical recovery.[8,10] With this in mind, the overt number of metastatic lesions amenable for resection is highly individualized to each patient. Although historically oligometastatic disease, defined as five or fewer lesions limited to three or fewer metastatic sites,[11] served as a guideline for possible resection of metastatic disease; currently instances exist that allow for resection of a greater number of metastatic lesions provided that the patient is an appropriate surgical candidate. For less-invasive ablative therapies, pulmonary function remains relevant, but with less stringent limitations than for surgery.[6] Beyond comorbidities, other patient-related factors include social support, compliance with medical advice, and emotional well-being.[12]

Optimal timing and sequencing of specific local intervention are imperative to ensure successful patient outcomes. In some circumstances, patients may benefit from upfront systemic treatment to reduce tumor volume, which may increase efficacy of subsequent radiation or ablative therapies[13] and/or reduce the amount of parenchyma required for resection. However, if tumors are particularly responsive to systemic therapy, small subcentimeter nodules may be difficult to localize, radiographically and intraoperatively. Thus, the interplay of systemic therapy with local therapies is an important component of the multidisciplinary discussion. Although limited studies have delved into this relationship between local and systemic therapies,[14] it is the subject of a current ongoing trial in lung-limited metastatic CRC.[15] There are a variety of modalities available for treatment of pulmonary metastases and numerous considerations guiding the applicability of each modality. Ultimately, for some patients, there may be an obvious best approach, whereas for others, there may be multiple reasonable strategies. Still yet for others, complete local control of pulmonary metastases may be best achieved with a hybrid approach. From here, we discuss the realm of surgery and identify the optimal timing and indications for its best use (or when to consider other strategies), with the overarching goal of highlighting the rationale for offering local therapy to patients with pulmonary metastatic disease.[6]

## NATURE OF THE PROBLEM/DIAGNOSIS

Conventional approaches to stage IV malignancies have historically centered around systemic therapy, aiming to address what has been perceived as a systemic state of disease. Recent years have seen the publication of numerous studies demonstrating the advantages of pulmonary metastasectomy, throughout a multitude of primary malignancies.[2,6,10,16–20] Although these promising results have been encouraging, there remains still a strong need for higher levels of evidence to further elucidate ideal candidates, because large, randomized control trials have been limited in number and scope.

Evidence supporting the use of pulmonary metastasectomy has become increasingly prevalent[2,10] such that its consideration of its use is recognized as standard of care by oncologic care teams. Ceppa and Tong describe pulmonary metastasectomy as the treatment of choice for patients with metastatic colon cancer, renal cell carcinoma, sarcomas, melanoma, and nonseminomatous germ cell tumors,[21] based on an abundance of retrospective data. A retrospective study published by

Blackmon and colleagues[9] showed that in 229 included patients with metastatic CRC, the median overall survival time was 70.1 months and the overall survival rate was 55.4%. A second study by Yun and colleagues[22] evaluating video-assisted thoracic surgery (VATS) for pulmonary metastases reviewed 173 patients retrospectively and found that 5-year survival rates were also greater than 50% (51.8%). Beyond this, a systematic review performed by Dickinson and Blackmon[23] found that on review of the literature in 2015, the pooled 5-year survival in patients who received pulmonary metastasectomy was 54%, whereas for patients with stage IV CRC median survival is 5 to 6 months.[24] This is further corroborated by a study by Corsini and colleagues[25] showing that there was a benefit from pulmonary metastasectomy regardless of laterality; however, the results were more pronounced in left-sided CRC because it was associated with a prolonged survival after pulmonary metastasectomy (hazard ratio [HR], 0.31; $P$ = 0.036) with a median survival time of 90 months.[25]

Beyond CRC, there exist data showing that patients with high-grade osteosarcoma who underwent resection of pulmonary metastases experienced 68.4% and 41%[20] 2- and 5-year postrelapse survival rates as compared with their counterparts in a nonsurgical group, which showed a 25.0% and 0% at 2 and 5 years, respectively.[20] Furthermore, a survival benefit was found in patients who achieved complete resection (32.3 months),[20] compared with those who underwent incomplete resections (14.4 months) and those not treated nonoperatively (13.8 months).[20] Also demonstrating benefits from pulmonary metastasectomy, a study by Gusho and colleagues[26] reviewed the Surveillance, Epidemiology, and End Results (SEER) database between 2010 and 2015 for patients with soft tissue sarcoma. The investigators compared 59 patients who underwent pulmonary metastasectomy with 202 patients who received medical management alone, finding the median disease-free survival in the metastasectomy group to be 32 months, compared with 20 months without resection ($P$ = 0.032), associated with an HR of 0.536 (95% confidence interval [CI], 0.33–0.85; $P$ = 0.008).[26] Similar results have been seen in renal cell carcinoma, as demonstrated by a systematic review by Ouzaid and colleagues.[27] This systematic review of 56 studies revealed a substantial gain in overall survival, with those undergoing pulmonary metastasectomy reaching median overall survivals of 36 to 142 months, compared with 8 to 27 months in patients who did not receive surgery.[27]

Although the preponderance of data in pulmonary metastatic disease is retrospective, there have been some important (yet limited) efforts previously attempted and currently underway to evaluate the benefit of pulmonary metastasectomy prospectively. The Pulmonary Metastasectomy versus Continued Active Monitoring in Colorectal Cancer (PulMICC) trial aimed to evaluate the additive benefit of surgery compared with active surveillance and closed prematurely in December 2016 without reaching the intended cohort size for randomization.[14] Subsequent analyses of the dataset demonstrated that patients in the control (nonoperative) group had better survival than had been previously assumed.[28] However, this study was limited by several factors, including that the majority of patients enrolled displayed highly favorable characteristics in terms of DFI and number of nodules, and that systemic agents were used by about one-half of the patients in both groups, yet were not standardized.[6] However, the authors should be praised for their important contributions to this space, setting a foundation for future prospective studies and important considerations as part of multidisciplinary discussion and informed consent.

It should be emphasized that one the goals and benefits of local therapy (including surgery, radiation, or ablative therapy) is to provide patients with potential freedom from systemic agents.[1] There currently exist little data to guide the interplay between systemic and local therapy for pulmonary metastatic disease, and practice patterns vary greatly among and even within institutions. Although completed clinical trials are lacking overall in the area of pulmonary metastasectomy, another multicenter trial is currently underway, under the umbrella of the Thoracic Surgery Oncology Group (TSOG),[15] examining multimodality management of risk-stratified patients with lung-limited metastatic CRC.[15] The primary goals of this study (TSOG 103) are to evaluate the additive benefit of chemotherapy on recurrence-free survival in low-risk patients undergoing metastasectomy, and to assess the role of surgery in prolonging overall survival among high-risk patients undergoing systemic therapy.

## ROLE OF SURGERY AS THE LOCAL THERAPY OF CHOICE FOR PULMONARY METASTASES

Although novel approaches to local therapy have emerged in recent years, surgery has been the mainstay of local therapy for pulmonary metastatic disease. The predominance of literature supporting this approach has been composed of retrospective reviews.[2,6,7,18,29] Although variability in patient populations and treatments has rendered a range of outcomes, in general, there is clear demonstration of improvement in prognosis for appropriately selected surgical patients.[1,6,16,25] Specifically, data show consistently and corroboratively that there is a particularly clear benefit for pulmonary metastasectomy in patients with a longer DFI, those patients without intrathoracic nodal disease, and patients with fewer total pulmonary nodules.

In reviewing evidence for the use of pulmonary metastasectomy, CRC has the greatest abundance of data, because it has been one of the earliest adopted and most frequent applications of strategy of surgical pulmonary metastasectomy. CRC is the most common extrathoracic malignancy to spread to the lungs, with up to 18% of patients developing metastatic disease.[30] A meta-analysis published by Gonzalez and colleagues[31] in 2013, reporting on nearly 3000 patients treated with metastasectomy, showed 5-year survival after resection of up to 68%. In this study, median DFI ranged 19 to 39 months, with longer DFI being associated with greater survival (HR for shorter DFI, 1.59).[31] Survival was also better among patients without intrathoracic nodal disease or multiple pulmonary nodules (HR for nodal involvement, 1.65; HR for >1 nodule, 2.04).[31] In 2016, Lumachi and colleagues[30] analyzed outcomes from 15 retrospective studies, describing a median 5-year survival of 45% after surgery, with some patient cohorts achieving 5-year survival of 72%.[30] This study, and a subsequent meta-analysis published in 2018, corroborated the findings that patients with the best prognosis following surgical resection were those with longer DFI, fewer pulmonary nodules, and absence of intrathoracic nodal disease.[30,32] Mutational status has also been shown to prognosticate outcome after resection of colorectal pulmonary metastases, with patients harboring mutant APC showing prolonged survival, whereas KRAS mutations have been associated with poorer outcomes after resection.[30,33] An additional prognostic factor for survival after pulmonary metastasectomy relates to the location of the primary CRC; patients with rectal tumors display shorter disease-free survival after pulmonary metastasectomy than those with colon tumors,[16] whereas patients whose initial tumors arose in the left-sided segments of colon (vs right-sided) tend to demonstrate the greatest survival benefit after lung resection.[25]

These findings of improved survival following pulmonary metastasectomy are corroborated in patients with metastatic sarcoma. Specifically, a review by Marulli and colleagues[34] demonstrated 5-year survival ranging from 15% to 51%, with tumor histology being particularly important to likelihood of survival after resection. Within this study, patients with osteosarcoma fared substantially better than those with soft tissue sarcoma.[34] As witnessed in the data for CRC, patients with sarcoma seem to have the best survival after pulmonary resection when they have fewer nodules, longer DFIs, and negative margins at the time of surgery.[17,34]

Surgery has been further found to be beneficial for pulmonary metastases in renal cell cancer and melanoma. For renal cell cancer, pulmonary metastasectomy has been shown to portend a 5-year survival in the range of 36% to 53%,[35,36] which is drastically improved over the durable complete responses approximating 10% of cases with comparable outcomes.[36,37] Similar benefit has been demonstrated in melanoma with surgical resection of pulmonary metastases conferring a 5-year survival rate of 21% as compared with an estimated 5% to 19% in medically managed patients with melanotic distant metastases.[19,35,38] As has been seen for CRC and sarcoma, patients with pulmonary metastatic disease from renal cell cancer and melanoma also seem to have greater benefit from metastasectomy when fewer lesions are present, DFI is longer, intrathoracic nodes are uninvolved, and surgical resection is complete.

Germ cell tumors are a rare phenomenon in the general population, but warrant mention because greater than 10% of patients who develop this disease develop pulmonary metastatic disease.[18] Pulmonary resection has been retrospectively studied in this patient population with excellent results, including 5-year survival ranging from 42% to 95%.[18] The timing of surgery, however, is of utmost importance because those who have completed a cisplatin-based chemotherapy with normalization of their tumor markers see the best results.[39]

## PATIENT SELECTION

When pulmonary metastatic disease is encountered, and surgical options are being considered there are a few criteria that ought to be considered to determine the treatment algorithm best suited for the patient. Specifically, all the pulmonary nodules must be resectable (or able to be addressed via hybrid approach with additional local therapy), the primary tumor must be controlled or controllable, the presence of extrathoracic disease must be controllable or controlled, an R0 resection is able to be achieved, and the patient has an acceptable preoperative risk.[6,8] If all these factors are met, then the patient is assessed as to whether

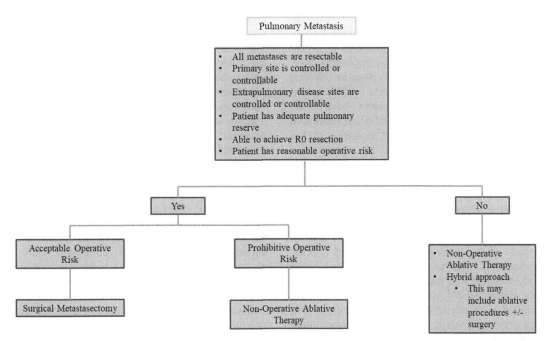

**Fig. 1.** Preoperative algorithm for surgical planning in instance of pulmonary metastases stemming from metastatic colon cancer, renal cell carcinoma, sarcomas, melanoma, and nonseminomatous germ cell tumors. Prohibitive operative risk as deemed by operative surgeon based on patient comorbidities. Nonoperative ablative therapy is inclusive of stereotactic ablative body radiation and transthoracic ablation techniques.

they have acceptable or prohibitive operative risk. In the setting of acceptable operative risk, metastasectomy should be performed.[6,8] For patients deemed to have prohibitive surgical risk, nonoperative techniques, such as radiofrequency ablation or stereotactic body radiation therapy, may be preferred (**Fig. 1**).[6] If the previously listed criteria is unable to be achieved, either a nonoperative approach or a hybrid approach (if acceptable operative risk is determined) may be considered.[6]

## TIMING OF SURGERY FOR PULMONARY METASTASES

The timing of pulmonary metastasectomy predominantly occurs following resolution or resection of the primary tumor and after the extrathoracic disease has been controlled.[40,41] There are select circumstances, however, that necessitate resection of the pulmonary metastases before the control of extrathoracic pathology. As a general principal, situations that would result in a significantly morbid procedure for the patient, such as extensive rectal cancer, would be best served by performing a pulmonary metastasectomy before resection of the primary cancer. Additionally, in circumstances where the primary tumor is confined to an extremity (ie, osteosarcoma), an index resection of the pulmonary metastases

before the amputation of the limb may be preferred.

## SURGICAL TECHNIQUE
### Surgical Approach

There exists ongoing debate regarding the best approach to pulmonary metastasectomy. To date, there are no randomized control trials exploring this topic; however, there are several case reports.[40–42] A review by Greenwood and West[29] offers reassuring albeit guarded evidence to support either VATS or open thoracotomy. Although there were high rates of complications, and longer hospital and chest tube durations[29] in patients undergoing thoracotomy for a variety of histologies, differences in baseline characteristics suggest the possibility of selection bias, limiting extrapolation of these data. Additionally, surgical margins were narrower in patients undergoing VATS metastasectomy,[29] but this did not demonstrate a survival difference between the two groups.

The optimal approach, thoracoscopy versus thoracotomy, is centered around the ability to find anticipated nodules (as evidenced on preoperative imaging) and the ability to remove additional nodules that may not have been identified on the preoperative scans.[43,44] Traditional dogma demonstrates superior ability to find nodules via thoracotomy and manual palpation.[45] Complicating the issue however, is that multiple investigators have failed to show differences in 5-year survival rates based on operative approach, likely because of widely disparate disease biology from within the patient cohorts.[10,29,43,46] Ultimately, the perioperative benefits have been shown to be approximately equal when enhanced recovery pathways are applied[47] and as such the exact operative approach should be deferred to the operating surgeon and based on the number of nodules, their exact anatomic locations, and other patient-specific factors.

A unique prospective investigation by Eckardt and Licht[43] reviewed the ability to identify pulmonary metastases identified on computed tomography (CT) through VATS and open thoracotomy. This prospective observer-blinded study evaluated 89 patients in whom 140 pulmonary metastases[43] were identified on CT and included a variety of primary malignancies. This was accomplished by the patients being taken to the operating room where they first underwent VATS during which digital palpation was attempted to identify the known nodule. Without resecting the metastasis, a new operating team completed a thoracotomy and similarly attempted to identify the nodules.[43] VATS was successful in identifying 122 (87%) of nodules,[43] whereas thoracotomy was able to identify all radiographically identified metastases. Beyond the metastases identified on imaging, 67 additional nodules were found, comprised of 22 (33%) secondary metastases, 43 (64%) benign lesions, and 2 (3%) primary lung malignancies.[43] In contrast, no extra tumors were identified via VATS. As a result of a significant proportion of the additional nodules being of malignant cause despite routine CT imaging (3 mm slice thickness), the authors concluded that VATS is inadequate for the management of pulmonary metastatic disease.[43] In a related review, Macherey and colleagues[44] reported an increased detection of nodules by manual palpation when compared with helical CT, although nearly half (48.5%) of these lesions were of benign cause. Conclusions from Macherey's report are limited, however, because the CT imaging studies included slice thickness in excess of 5 mm, up to and including 10 mm.[44] Despite the increased detection rates associated with thoracotomy, survival rates do not differ when considering patients undergoing thoracotomy versus VATS resections.[35]

The selection of surgical approach should also be weighed with the risk of postoperative complications. Greenwood and West[29] found the length of hospital stay and chest tube duration to be shorter among patients undergoing VATS resection, although as previously stated selection bias may limit the generalizability of these data. The authors were unable to demonstrate survival differences between the two surgical groups, but postoperative complication events were more common in patients undergoing thoracotomy[29] and as a result, as highlighted previously, the preferred operative approach should be tailored to patient- and tumor-specific characteristics.

For patients with bilateral disease, simultaneous metastasectomy is a safe option as compared with a staged approach. A treatment algorithm similar to that listed previously should be considered. A study performed by Feldman and colleagues[48] demonstrated the advantages of a simultaneous operation as compared with a staged approach, including a shorter hospital stay (3 vs 8 days; $P < 0.001$) and a shorter operative time when compared with the sum of both procedures (156 vs 235.5 minutes; $P < 0.001$).[48] This produces advantages for the patient and the hospital system including lower cost and fewer resources required.

### Extent of Resection

In determining the extent of the resection for pulmonary metastasectomy, a focus should be placed on preserving the maximal amount of parenchyma as is feasible. This focus differs from the management of primary lung cancer.[6,49] The focus of parenchyma conservation is driven by the frequent need for resection of multiple nodules, the potential need for future resections and/or ablative therapy, the lack of data demonstrating benefit in more extensive resections, and the expectation of less postoperative morbidity.[1,46,50] Most commonly, a stapled wedge resection is performed, whereas more extensive anatomic resections, such as a lobectomy, are reserved for larger tumors, central tumors, or the presence of multiple metastases within a given lobe.[10,32,49,50] By using this technique, postoperative morbidity is minimized. In comparison with a stapled wedge, segmentectomy may also have superior overall and disease-free survival according to some reports.[10,50]

In assessing the optimal margin length, a recent publication by Nelson and colleagues[51] demonstrated that a margin at least half the size of the local tumor resulted in a local recurrence risk of less than 11% within 2 years. To determine this figure, the authors of that publication evaluated 1-cm, 2-cm, and 4-cm tumors. For 1-cm tumors, the risk of local recurrence within 2 years was 11.08% (95% CI, 5.39%–16.43%)[51] provided a

0.5-cm margin was obtained and 7.45% (95% CI, 2.77%–11.90%)[51] provided a 1-cm margin was obtained. For a 2-cm tumor the risk of local recurrence was 11.09% (95% CI, 4.44%–17.28%)[51] with a 1-cm margin, and 4.97% (95% CI, 0.00%–10.22%)[51] with a 2-cm margin. For 4-cm tumors local recurrence was 23.76% (95% CI, 0.54%–55.43%)[51] with a 1-cm margin, and 11.11% (95% CI, 0.00%–23.76%) with a 2-cm marigin.[51]

Several authors have suggested when considering a pneumonectomy during the preoperative planning stage for pulmonary metastasis, that such extent of needed resection should be considered a strong contraindication for surgical intervention.[6,7,52,53] This recommendations stems from the known elevated risks associated with pneumonectomy, with up to a 19% postoperative mortality risk.[52] However, for patients with a solitary central tumor after a prolonged DFI and that have demonstrated disease stability and absence of disease elsewhere,[7,10] pneumonectomy may be considered by some experienced surgeons.[52] For more peripheral disease, however, given the lack of evidence, completeness of resection continues to be cited as the most important consideration for any metastasectomy. In sum, a lung-sparing approach has been shown to be noninferior and has added benefit of preserving lung parenchyma in the event the patient needs future pulmonary resections, with the exception of if it were to leave positive margins.[7,10]

### Lymphadenectomy

The role of lymphadenectomy when performing pulmonary metastasectomy remains a debatable topic. The presence of intrathoracic nodal disease portends a worse prognosis, and there has not been data supportive of a clear survival benefit, although the data are limited by heterogeneity of the study populations.[54] Thus, the utility of lymphadenectomy is unclear because it may aid in obtaining a more accurate prognosis, although that seems to be of little therapeutic benefit if the presence of nodal disease is known preoperatively.

### Reoperative Resection

Because of the systemic nature of disease that is encountered with pulmonary metastases, repeat metastasectomy is sometimes required. Importantly, recent investigators have demonstrated similar, if not improved, efficacy of repeat pulmonary metastasectomy in the setting of recurrence. A systematic review by Ambrogi and colleagues[55] reviewed 120 papers meeting relevant criteria and found that 5-year survival rates after repeat lung resection were approximately 50%, ultimately

concluding that reoperative metastasectomy is worthwhile when lesions are resectable and perioperative risk is low.[55] Additionally, a retrospective multicenter trial performed by Kruger and colleagues[56] found that, among 64 patients undergoing repeat pulmonary metastasectomies for colorectal, 5-year survival rates of 50.9% were demonstrated for second resections, 74.4% after third resections, 83.3% after fourth resections, and 60.0% after the fifth. Regarding the perioperative outcomes of repeat metastasectomy, Mills[57] studied patients undergoing three or greater pulmonary resections for metastatic disease. Outcomes of this study importantly revealed that overall complication rates were similar irrespective of the number of resections performed. The author did note, however, an increase in wound complications between the second and third procedures (0.9% vs 6.8%; $P = 0.02$), and a trend toward incremental increase in the incidence of prolonged air leaks.[57] Ultimately, the author concluded that in appropriately selected patients, repeat pulmonary metastasectomy is a safe and feasible treatment modality in the presence of disease recurrence.[57]

## FUTURE OF LOCAL MANAGEMENT FOR PULMONARY METASTATIC DISEASE

The future of the role of pulmonary metastasectomy may lie in assessing the genomic and biomarker status of patients. As an example, for patients with CRC the mutational status may affect the likelihood of prolonged survival after metastasectomy and those with APC mutations may be best advised to undergo resection.[15] As the fund of knowledge continues to grow, clinicians may be able to optimize recommendations for individual patients. The aim is that as TSOG 103 delineates the interplay of various treatment modalities and examines the changes in circulating tumor DNA after surgical resection or chemotherapy, the groundwork can be developed regarding biomarker status that can guide the treatment choice for individual patients.

Additionally, as one looks toward the future management of pulmonary metastatic disease, further exploration into options for local therapy for patients with extended criteria must be considered. Conclusive evidence comparing local control of surgery with ablative therapy within the lung is lacking; however, survival outcomes in a systematic review of CRC, renal cell cancer, and sarcoma treated with percutaneous ablation techniques provided 5-year survival rates of 50%, 57%, and 34%, respectively, suggesting that such strategies may be reasonable for small (<2 cm) centrally located tumors may be noninferior for patients who are not surgical candidates.[58] Moreover, it will be of particular benefit to formulate consensus strategies regarding the role of surgery when R0 resection cannot be achieved. Within this patient population, there may be limited but important criteria for which resection of a tumor may be beneficial. First, surgery may be appropriate in patients who have heterogeneity among their tumors, such that there is a dominant mass (or masses) growing more rapidly or causing more local symptoms. Also, hybrid approaches may be warranted for patients with extensive disease or with combination of lesions with varying ease of resectability. For example, smaller, deeper lesions may be more amenable to ablation because of the challenges in identifying such lesions intraoperatively and sparing parenchyma, whereas more superficial lesions may be more appropriate for surgical resection.

It is exceedingly clear that as the armamentarium of systemic agents continues to grow in number and efficacy, the population of patients living for extended periods with stage IV malignancies will continue to expand. As such, more patients may survive to the development of pulmonary metastases and to the point of multiple recurrences of pulmonary metastases. Through these circumstances, the ability to provide hybrid approaches that optimize all multidisciplinary tools to address pulmonary parenchymal disease will be pivotal to prolonging DFIs, patient quality of life (via freedom from systemic agents), and it is hoped, survival.

The decision to pursue surgery, ultimately, must be individualized on a patient-by-patient basis, and a collaborative decision should be made with input from the patients, their families, and the multidisciplinary oncology team.

## CLINICS CARE POINTS

- Historically, conventional approaches to pulmonary metastases have surrounded the use of systemic therapy; however, ample data suggest that surgical resection may provide improved overall survival to carefully selected patients.
- One of the goals and benefits of local therapy, which includes surgery, radiation, or ablative therapy, is to provide patients with freedom from systemic agents.
- Pulmonary metastasectomy, as a central tenant of local therapy, has demonstrated the most substantial benefits in patients with longer disease-free intervals (DFI), those

patients without intrathoracic nodal disease, and patients with fewer total pulmonary nodules.

- Regarding patient selection, we recommend the following considerations: patients must have acceptable operative risk, primary tumors must be controlled or controllable, and all pulmonary lesions must be resectable or amenable to hybrid multimodal local therapy.
- In most cases, pulmonary metastasectomy follows resolution or resection of the primary tumor and control of extrathoracic disease. Select circumstances, such as instances that portend significant morbidity to the patient, may be better served by upfront pulmonary metastasectomy.
- Optimal surgical approach, open thoracotomy versus minimally invasive surgery, is deferred to the operating surgeon.
- When deciding between open thoracotomy and video-assisted thoracic surgery (VATS), studies suggest VATS has shorter hospital stay and chest tube durations but this may be at the expense of finding additional lesions, which are more easily identified via manual palpation during thoracotomy.
- For patients with bilateral disease, simultaneous metastasectomy represents a safe option in well-selected patients compared with a staged approach.
- In determining extent of resection, focus should be placed on preserving the maximal amount of parenchyma; thus, wedge resections are preferred over anatomic resections when feasible.
- To determine optimal margin length, ideal margins should equal at least half of pulmonary nodule diameter, when feasible.
- Pneumonectomy should be considered a contraindication to resection except in cases with a solitary central tumor, a prolonged DFI, and demonstration of disease stability and absence of disease elsewhere.
- The role of lymphadenectomy remains unclear, because it may provide benefit in obtaining a more accurate prognosis, but without significant therapeutic benefit in the instance of known nodal involvement preoperatively.
- Repeat pulmonary metastasectomy is a safe and feasible treatment modality in the presence of disease recurrence.
- Future trials are in need, with current prospective trials seeking to examine multimodal management of risk-stratified patients with lung-limited metastases.

## DISCLOSURE

No conflicts of interests to disclose. This work is supported by the Mason Family Research Fund.

## REFERENCES

1. Corsini EM, Antonoff MB. Is pulmonary metastasectomy effective in prolonging survival?. In: Ferguson MK, editor. Difficult decisions in thoracic surgery: an evidence-based approach. New York, NY: Springer International Publishing; 2020. p. 279–89.

2. Cheung FP-Y, Alam NZ, Wright GM. The past, present and future of pulmonary metastasectomy: a review article. Ann Thorac Cardiovasc Surg 2019; 25(3):129–41.

3. Jamil A, Kasi A. Lung metastasis. StatPearls. In: StatPearls Publishing Copyright ©2022. Tampa, FL: StatPearls Publishing LLC; 2022.

4. Petrella F, Diotti C, Rimessi A, et al. Pulmonary metastasectomy: an overview. J Thorac Dis 2017;9(Suppl 12):S1291–8.

5. Schweiger T, Lang G, Klepetko W, et al. Prognostic factors in pulmonary metastasectomy: spotlight on molecular and radiological markers. Eur J Cardio Thorac Surg 2014;45(3):408–16.

6. Antonoff MB, Sofocleous CT, Callstrom MR, et al. The roles of surgery, stereotactic radiation, and ablation for treatment of pulmonary metastases. J Thorac Cardiovasc Surg 2022;163(2):495–502.

7. Handy JR, Bremner RM, Crocenzi TS, et al. Expert consensus document on pulmonary metastasectomy. Ann Thorac Surg 2019;107(2):631–49.

8. Erhunmwunsee L, Tong BC. Preoperative evaluation and indications for pulmonary metastasectomy. Thorac Surg Clin 2016;26(1):7–12.

9. Blackmon SH, Stephens EH, Correa AM, et al. Predictors of recurrent pulmonary metastases and survival after pulmonary metastasectomy for colorectal cancer. Ann Thorac Surg 2012;94(6): 1802–9.

10. Nichols FC. Pulmonary metastasectomy: role of pulmonary metastasectomy and type of surgery. Curr Treat Options Oncol 2014;15(3):465–75.

11. Chandy ETJ, Saxby I IJ, Pang JW, et al. The multidisciplinary management of oligometastases from colorectal cancer: a narrative review. Ann Palliat Med 2020;10(5):5988–6001.

12. Brunelli AMD, Socci LMD, Refai MMD, et al. Quality of life before and after major lung resection for lung cancer: a prospective follow-up analysis. Ann Thorac Surg 2007;84(2):410–6.

13. Chua TC, Thornbury K, Saxena A, et al. Radiofrequency ablation as an adjunct to systemic chemotherapy for colorectal pulmonary metastases. Cancer 2010;116(9):2106–14.

14. Treasure T, Farewell V, Macbeth F, et al. Pulmonary metastasectomy versus continued active monitoring in colorectal cancer (PulMiCC): a multicentre randomised clinical trial. Trials 2019;20(1):718.

15. Antonoff MB. Registered Clinical Trial: Chemotherapy and/or metastasectomy in treating patients with metastatic colorectal adenocarcinoma with lung metastases 2022;NCT03599752. https:// clinicaltrials.gov/ct2/show/NCT03599752.

16. Cho JHMD, Hamaji MMD, Allen MSMD, et al. The prognosis of pulmonary metastasectomy depends on the location of the primary colorectal cancer. Ann Thorac Surg 2014;98(4):1231–7.

17. Chudgar NPMD, Brennan MFMD, Munhoz RRMD, et al. Pulmonary metastasectomy with therapeutic intent for soft-tissue sarcoma. J Thorac Cardiovasc Surg 2017;154(1):319–30.e1.

18. Farazdaghi A, Vaughn DJ, Singhal S. Pulmonary metastasectomy for germ cell tumors. Ann Thorac Cardiovasc Surg 2019;ra.19–00070. https://doi.org/ 10.5761/atcs.ra.19-00070.

19. Hanna TP, Chauvin C, Miao Q, et al. Clinical outcomes after pulmonary metastasectomy for melanoma: a population-based study. Ann Thorac Surg 2018;106(6):1675–81.

20. Liu Z, Yin J, Zhou Q, et al. Survival after pulmonary metastasectomy for relapsed osteosarcoma. J Thorac Cardiovasc Surg 2022;163(2):469–79.e8.

21. Doty JR, Vricella LA, Yang SC, et al. Johns Hopkins textbook of cardiothoracic surgery. 2nd edition. New York, NY: McGraw-Hill's AccessMedicine. McGraw Hill Medical; 2007.

22. Yun JS, Kim E, Na KJ, et al. Thoracoscopic pulmonary metastasectomy in metastatic colorectal cancer: surgical outcomes and prognostic factors. Thorac Cancer 2021;12(19):2537–43.

23. Dickinson KJ, Blackmon SH. Results of pulmonary resection: colorectal carcinoma. Thorac Surg Clin 2016;26(1):41–7.

24. Labianca R, Beretta GD, Kildani B, et al. Colon cancer. Crit Rev Oncol Hematol 2010;74(2):106–33.

25. Corsini EM, Mitchell KG, Correa A, et al. Effect of primary colorectal cancer tumor location on survival after pulmonary metastasectomy. J Thorac Cardiovasc Surg 2021;162(1):296–305.

26. Gusho CA, Seder CW, Lopez-Hisijos N, et al. Pulmonary metastasectomy in bone and soft tissue sarcoma with metastasis to the lung. Interact Cardiovasc Thorac Surg 2021;33(6):879–84.

27. Ouzaid I, Capitanio U, Staehler M, et al. Surgical metastasectomy in renal cell carcinoma: a systematic review. Eur Urol Oncol 2019;2(2):141–9.

28. Milosevic M, Edwards J, Tsang D, et al. Pulmonary metastasectomy in colorectal cancer: updated analysis of 93 randomized patients – control survival is much better than previously assumed. Colorectal Dis 2020;22(10):1314–24.

29. Greenwood A, West D. Is a thoracotomy rather than thoracoscopic resection associated with improved survival after pulmonary metastasectomy? Interact Cardiovasc Thorac Surg 2013;17(4):720–4.

30. Lumachi F, Mazza F, Del Conte A, et al. Factors affecting survival in patients with pulmonary metastases from colorectal cancer with previously resected liver metastases who underwent lung metastasectomy. Ann Oncol 2015;26:i45.

31. Gonzalez M, Poncet A, Combescure C, et al. Risk factors for survival after lung metastasectomy in colorectal cancer patients: a systematic review and meta-analysis. Ann Surg Oncol 2012;20(2):572–9.

32. Zabaleta J, Iida T, Falcoz PE, et al. Individual data meta-analysis for the study of survival after pulmonary metastasectomy in colorectal cancer patients: a history of resected liver metastases worsens the prognosis. Eur J Surg Oncol 2018;44(7):1006–12.

33. Corsini EM, Mitchell KG, Mehran RJ, et al. Colorectal cancer mutations are associated with survival and recurrence after pulmonary metastasectomy. J Surg Oncol 2019;120(4):729–35.

34. Marulli G, Mammana M, Comacchio G, et al. Survival and prognostic factors following pulmonary metastasectomy for sarcoma. J Thorac Dis 2017; 9(Suppl 12):S1305–15.

35. Ripley RT, Downey RJ. Pulmonary metastasectomy. J Surg Oncol 2014;109(1):42–6.

36. Zhao Y, Li J, Li C, et al. Prognostic factors for overall survival after lung metastasectomy in renal cell cancer patients: a systematic review and meta-analysis. Int J Surg 2017;41:70–7.

37. Marincola FM, White DE, Wise AP, et al. Combination therapy with interferon alfa-2a and interleukin-2 for the treatment of metastatic cancer. J Clin Oncol May 1995;13(5):1110–22.

38. Sandru A, Voinea S, Panaitescu E, et al. Survival rates of patients with metastatic malignant melanoma. J Med Life 2014;7(4):572–6.

39. Krege S, Beyer J, Souchon R, et al. European consensus conference on diagnosis and treatment of germ cell cancer: a report of the second meeting of the European Germ Cell Cancer Consensus Group (EGCCCG): Part II. Eur Urol 2008;53(3):497–513.

40. Krüger M, Schmitto JD, Wiegmann B, et al. Optimal timing of pulmonary metastasectomy: is a delayed operation beneficial or counterproductive? Eur J Surg Oncol 2014;40(9):1049–55.

41. Yamada K, Ozawa D, Onozato R, et al. Optimal timing for the resection of pulmonary metastases in patients with colorectal cancer. Medicine (Baltim) 2020;99(9): e19144.

42. Ahmed G, Zamzam M, Kamel A, et al. Effect of timing of pulmonary metastasis occurrence on the outcome of metastasectomy in osteosarcoma patients. J Pediatr Surg 2019;54(4):775–9.

43. Eckardt JMD, Licht PBMDP. Thoracoscopic or open surgery for pulmonary metastasectomy: an observer blinded study. Ann Thorac Surg 2014;98(2):466–70.

44. Macherey S, Doerr F, Heldwein M, et al. Is manual palpation of the lung necessary in patients undergoing pulmonary metastasectomy? Interact Cardiovasc Thorac Surg 2016;22(3):351–9.

45. Cerfolio RJ, McCarty T, Bryant AS. Non-imaged pulmonary nodules discovered during thoracotomy for metastasectomy by lung palpation. Eur J Cardio Thorac Surg 2009;35(5):786–91.

46. Lo Faso F, Solaini L, Lembo R, et al. Thoracoscopic lung metastasectomies: a 10-year, single-center experience. Surg Endosc 2013;27(6):1938–44.

47. Van Haren RM, Mehran RJ, Mena GE, et al. Enhanced recovery decreases pulmonary and cardiac complications after thoracotomy for lung cancer. Ann Thorac Surg 2018;106(1):272–9.

48. Feldman HA, Zhou N, Antonoff MB, et al. Simultaneous versus staged resections for bilateral pulmonary metastases. J Surg Oncol 2021;123(7):1633–9.

49. McKenna JRJ. Surgical management of primary lung cancer. Semin Oncol 2007;34(3):250–5.

50. Phillips JD, Hasson RM. Surgical management of colorectal lung metastases. J Surg Oncol 2019; 119(5):629–35.

51. Nelson DB, Tayob N, Mitchell KG, et al. Surgical margins and risk of local recurrence after wedge resection of colorectal pulmonary metastases. J Thorac Cardiovasc Surg 2019;157(4):1648–55.

52. Strand TE, Rostad H, Damhuis RA, et al. Risk factors for 30-day mortality after resection of lung cancer and prediction of their magnitude. Thorax 2007;62(11):991–7.

53. Treasure T, Dunning J, Williams NR, et al. Lung metastasectomy for colorectal cancer: the impression of benefit from uncontrolled studies was not supported in a randomized controlled trial. J Thorac Cardiovasc Surg 2022;163(2):486–90.

54. Seebacher GMD, Decker SMD, Fischer JRMD, et al. Unexpected lymph node disease in resections for pulmonary metastases. Ann Thorac Surg 2015;99(1):231–6.

55. Ambrogi V, Tamburrini A, Tajé R. Results of redo pulmonary metastasectomy. J Thorac Dis 2021;13(4): 2669–85.

56. Krüger M, Franzke K, Rajab TK, et al. Outcome of repeat pulmonary metastasectomy. Adv Exp Med Biol 2021;1335:37–44.

57. Mills AC. Repeat pulmonary metastasectomy: third operations and beyond. Ann Thorac Surg 2022. https://doi.org/10.1016/j.athoracsur.2022.07.025.

58. Nguyenhuy M, Xu Y, Maingard J, et al. A systematic review and meta-analysis of patient survival and disease recurrence following percutaneous ablation of pulmonary metastasis. Cardiovasc Intervent Radiol 2022;45(8):1102–13.

# Current Management of Carcinoid Tumor
## When Is a Wedge Enough?

Micaela Langille Collins, MD, MPH[a], Olugbenga Okusanya, MD[b],*

**KEYWORDS**

- Bronchopulmonary carcinoid • Pulmonary neuroendocrine tumor • Anatomic resection
- Sublobar resection • Segmental resection • Wedge resection • Segmentectomy

**KEY POINTS**

- Bronchopulmonary carcinoid tumors are low-to-intermediate-grade, well-differentiated tumors of neuroendocrine origin.
- Their rarity has led to a relative paucity of available data and large-scale studies to delineate optimal treatment of these tumors.
- The mainstay of treating localized or locoregional disease is surgical resection and consensus guidelines recommend anatomic resection for stage I to IIIA disease.
- Recent publications have challenged this notion and suggested that a wedge resection may be sufficient for small, early-stage, low-grade bronchopulmonary carcinoids.
- As sublobar resections are becoming standard for the treatment of other lung malignancies, it is most reasonable to perform an anatomic resection for the treatment of undifferentiated or carcinoid lung nodules.

## INTRODUCTION AND EPIDEMIOLOGY

Bronchopulmonary carcinoid tumors are well-differentiated neuroendocrine neoplasms comprising approximately 1% to 2% of all lung malignancies, with a yearly incidence of 0.2 to 2/100 000 population/year.[1] Their incidence has increased over the past 30 years, though this is thought to be secondary to increased detection of early lesions.[2] Carcinoids are subdivided by histologic features into typical carcinoids (TC) and atypical carcinoids (AC) based on the World Health Organization Classification of Lung Tumors 2021[3] (**Table 1**). Other varieties of pulmonary neuroendocrine tumors, historically referred to as large-cell neuroendocrine carcinoma and small-cell lung cancer, are poorly differentiated and tend to be high grade.[3–5] Bronchopulmonary carcinoids are distinct entities from high-grade neuroendocrine tumors and do not share with them any genetic or epidemiological traits.[1,4] TC outnumber AC approximately 8:1 and are usually sporadic, though rarely may be familial or associated with multiple endocrine neoplasia 1 (MEN1).[1,4] In addition, TC appear to have no association with smoking, and AC have only a small association.[3,4,6,7] Both typical and AC have a slight female predominance, again in contrast to other lung malignancies.[3,4,6,7] Diagnosis is usually in the fourth to sixth decade of life and tends to be earlier in cases of TC when compared with AC.[1,4,5,8] Both typical and AC carry a favorable prognosis, with ~87% to 92% 5-year survival for TC, and 56% to 85% 5-year survival for AC, depending on grade, stage at diagnosis.[5,7,9,10] TC are indolent, less likely to recur, and less likely to metastasize.[5] AC are more aggressive and recur in a quarter of patients.[5] They are more likely to metastasize and

[a] Department of Surgery, Thomas Jefferson University Hospital, 1015 Walnut Street, Suite 620, Philadelphia, PA 19107, USA; [b] Division of Thoracic Surgery, Department of Surgery, Thomas Jefferson University Hospital, 211 South 9th Street, Suite 300, Philadelphia, PA 19107, USA
* Corresponding author.
*E-mail address:* Olugbenga.okusanya@jefferson.edu
Twitter: @micaelacollins (M.L.C.); @okusanyamd (O.O.)

Thorac Surg Clin 33 (2023) 159–164
https://doi.org/10.1016/j.thorsurg.2023.01.008
1547-4127/23/© 2023 Elsevier Inc. All rights reserved.

**Table 1**
**World Health Organization classification of carcinoid tumors**

|  | Typical Carcinoid | Atypical Carcinoid |
|---|---|---|
| Mitosis (per mm$^2$) | <2 | 2 to 10 |
| Necrosis | Absent | Absent or punctate foci |

*Data from* Refs.[10,11]

more frequently associated with carcinoid syndrome than TC, although the overall incidence of carcinoid syndrome at the time of diagnosis is extremely low (1% to 5%, most often when metastatic spread to the liver is present).[1,5] Cushing's syndrome, seen in 1% to 6% of patients, is associated with TC with localized spread.[1,5,10] The most common sites for metastatic disease are liver, bone, and mediastinal lymph nodes.[1]

## CLASSIFICATION AND STAGING

Classification of neuroendocrine tumors is an evolving process. The pathologic features and thresholds used to classify carcinoids, as well as differentiating typical from atypical carcinoid have changed over the past 20 years. The most recent categorization in the World Health Organization Classification of Lung Tumors in 2021 groups all pulmonary neuroendocrine malignancies into one category, neuroendocrine neoplasms.[12] This is subdivided into neuroendocrine tumors (carcinoids) and neuroendocrine carcinomas (small cell lung cancer and large cell neuroendocrine carcinoma). The latter two are considered grade 3 neoplasms. Typical and atypical carcinoids correspond to grade 1 and grade 2 neuroendocrine tumors, respectively.[12] The primary criteria used to differentiate between typical and atypical carcinoid is mitotic count, reported in number per 2 mm$^2$ as well as the presence or absence of necrosis.[12,13] Ki-67, a measure of cellular proliferation, may be a useful metric by which to differentiate between carcinoids and high-grade neuroendocrine tumors in small or crushed cellular samples.[1,3,12] However, data have been conflicting on its prognostic utility for differentiating between typical and atypical carcinoid and no formal cut-offs have been established, though an index of >30% is usually seen in neuroendocrine carcinomas.[1,10,12] It remains a suggestion rather than a formal component of classification.[11]

Bronchopulmonary carcinoid tumors are pathologically and clinically staged using the International Association for the Study of Lung Cancer (IASLC) tumor, node, metastasis (TNM) classification, in concordance with other forms of lung cancer.[1,2,10,14,15] More than 80% of carcinoids are diagnosed at stage I or stage II.[10]

## DIAGNOSIS

Bronchopulmonary carcinoids may present as central or peripheral lesions. The majority of typical pulmonary carcinoids are centrally located, while atypical carcinoids tend to be peripheral.[16] Peripheral lesions are often asymptomatic and found incidentally on routine or screening radiographs or computed tomography (CT) scans.[5,16] Central lesions may be associated with atelectatic changes, cough, repeated upper respiratory tract infections, and dyspnea secondary to endoluminal obstruction.[4] TC are highly vascular, and hemoptysis may be a presenting symptom, though approximately one-third to half of the patients are asymptomatic at the time of diagnosis.[1,6,7]

Initial workup should begin with a chest radiograph, though findings may be non-specific, and contrast-enhanced CT scan is the recommended diagnostic modality of choice.[1,15,16] On chest radiographs, carcinoids appear as well-defined, ovoid, or round lesions.[1,16] Calcification can be present, especially in cases of AC.[16] Central carcinoids appear as smooth hilar or perihilar masses, and evidence of airway obstruction (air trapping and atelectasis) may be present on CT.[1,5] Cross-sectional imaging of the abdomen should also be performed, given the propensity of carcinoids to metastasize to the liver.[1,15] Additional nuclear imaging techniques such as somatostatin receptor (SSTR)-PET/CT, SSTR-PET/MRI, or F-fluorodeoxygenase (FDG)-PET may be considered, but the utility of these modalities may be limited and a full discussion of the controversies associated with their diagnostic utility is beyond the scope of this article.[1,10,15,16] It is widely agreed upon that diagnosis and workup of bronchopulmonary carcinoids should be undertaken at a specialized care center and with a multidisciplinary team given the disease's rarity.[1,4–6,10]

The European Society of Medical Oncology (ESMO) and the European Neuroendocrine Tumor Society (ENTS) recommend flexible bronchoscopy and biopsy for all centrally located carcinoids, whereas the National Comprehensive Cancer Network (NCCN) recommends bronchoscopy only if clinically indicated.[1,10,15] CT-guided or endobronchial endoscopic ultrasound (EBUS) is recommended for the biopsy of peripheral lesions.[1,10] However, biopsy may not yield sufficient tissue for diagnosis, and it can be exceedingly difficult to discern typical from atypical carcinoid, even on intraoperative frozen sample.[4,5] Formal diagnosis may not be able to be made until after surgical excision of the lesion.[6]

## TREATMENT

Surgical resection remains the treatment of choice for TC and AC stage I to IIIA and will be discussed in detail in the sections below. The role of adjuvant chemotherapy or chemoradiation remains a hotly debated topic. Several large-scale studies examining adjuvant treatment have failed to show a statistically significant survival benefit and in fact were associated with worse outcomes in some patient subsets.[17–20] ESMO, ENETS, and NCCN are in relative concordance with their recommendations: adjuvant chemotherapy, radiation, or treatment with somatostatin analogs is not recommended for stage I or stage II AC, or for stage I to III TC.[1,10,15,18] The NCCN additionally states that adjuvant cytotoxic chemotherapy may be considered in a patient with advanced AC disease (stage III), whereas ENETS advises chemotherapy and/or radiation may be considered in cases of stage III, node-positive AC disease only.[1,15] ESMO recommends adjuvant therapy only in patients with a high risk of relapse and stresses an individualized approach to therapy.[10]

### Surgical Resection

Surgery is the standard of care for the treatment of bronchopulmonary carcinoid and is often curative. However, recommendations regarding the degree of resection have changed over time and vary depending on the tumor subtype and location. The rarity of AC has made their study extremely difficult, and there is insufficient data available to make subtype-specific treatment recommendations.[21,22] The remainder of this article will focus on surgical treatment of TC only.

Current guidelines indicate that for early-stage, centrally located TC, bronchosplastic procedures or sleeve resections should be performed to ensure oncologic resection and sufficient lymphadenectomy for staging purposes while preserving as much lung parenchyma as possible.[1,5,10,23,24] Rea and colleagues[24] in their retrospective analysis of 252 patients who received surgery for bronchopulmonary carcinoids at a single center in Italy over the course of 36 years showed an evolution in surgical approach. Patients who received treatment in the last 15 years of the study (1990 to 2005) were less likely to undergo pneumonectomy, and more likely to receive a parenchymal-sparing resection. They attribute this to improved surgical technique as well as data supporting the non-inferiority of parenchymal-sparing resections with respect to operative risk and disease recurrence.[24] As with other forms of lung cancer, pneumonectomy should be avoided whenever possible.

For many years, lobectomy was considered the only acceptable procedure of choice for peripheral TC. The popularity of segmental resection has gained traction in the past decade, with large-scale studies deomonstrating its non-inferiority to lobectomy with respect to overall survival in select cases of early-stage non-small cell lung cancer.[25,26] Similarly, segmental resection has gained popularity as an acceptable treatment of TC tumors. Afoke and colleagues[21] performed a best evidence topic review of the available literature to determine if sublobar resection (segmentectomy or wedge resection) is equivalent to lobectomy in terms of operative morbidity and mortality, long-term survival and disease recurrence in patients with peripheral carcinoid tumors. They found that sublobar resection with lymphadenectomy may be sufficient for patients with TC, though they note that high-quality studies are needed to assess morbidity, survival, and disease recurrence.[21] Two additional retrospective analyses of bronchopulmonary carcinoids from the Surveillance Epidemiology and End Results Registry (SEER) concluded that after multivariate analysis, sublobar resection was non-inferior to lobectomy with respect to the overall survival of patients with TC.[27,28] Limitations of these studies are inherent to the database used and include the fact that histologic criteria for carcinoid were changed in 1998, and the database changed staging criteria to the TMN model in 2004. A more recent analysis using SEER data from patients with cT1-3N0M0 peripheral disease from 2000 to 2015 similarly concluded that sublobar resection was not associated with any significant difference in recurrence-free or overall survival when compared with lobectomy.[29]

Current NCCN, ESMO, and ENET guidelines recommend anatomic resection (segmentectomy or lobectomy) with mediastinal lymph node dissection for treatment of stage I to IIIA TC.[1,10,15] All guidelines stress the importance of lymph node sampling to ensure proper disease staging. What constitutes adequate lymph node sampling is not specified by the NCCN or ESMO, though ENETS recommends adherence to the IASLC guideline of six nodal stations, three of which should be mediastinal, and one of which should be subcarinal.[1]

## DISCUSSION: WHEN IS A WEDGE ENOUGH?

Many of the existing studies looking at whether the degree of resection impacts outcomes for patients with early-stage TC tumors compared sublobar resection (segmentectomy or wedge resection) to lobectomy, and found that degree of resection does not impact overall survival. These results, and the indolent nature of TC, have led some groups to question whether an anatomic resection is necessary at all in early-stage disease.

Rahouma and colleagues[30] used the SEER database to compare overall and cancer-specific survival of patients with carcinoid tumors who had an anatomic resection (segmentectomy or lobectomy) versus a wedge resection. For patients with TC, they found no difference in overall survival or cancer-specific survival between the two groups. Yan and colleagues[31] used the SEER database from 2004 to 2015 to compare wedge resection and segmental resection for patients with TC. After propensity matching, they found no difference in overall survival at 5 and 10 years between the two groups. These results run contrary to the findings of Filosso and colleagues.[32] Using the European Society of Thoracic Surgeons Neuroendocrine Tumors of the Lung Working Group (ESTS NETs-WG) database, they set out to compare overall survival between three groups: patients with stage I TC who received a lobectomy, a segmentectomy, or a wedge resection. They found a lower 5-year survival rate in patients who received a wedge resection (82% vs 96% for lobectomy and 95% for segmentectomy) though note that patients who received a wedge resection tended to be significantly older and with worse underlying medical conditions, both attributes which may have impacted overall survival as well as choice of procedure.[32]

Two more recent studies have been published with conflicting results. Bachman and colleagues[33] performed a retrospective analysis of 821 patients with cT1N0M0 TC tumors from the NCDB years 2010 to 2016. They found that patients who received a wedge resection had similar overall survival to those who underwent segmentectomy, a finding that was preserved after propensity matching.[33] The authors argue that wedge resections are safer than anatomic resections with respect to perioperative morbidity and mortality, citing a 2014 Society of Thoracic Surgery (STS) database review,[34] though in their study there was no difference in 90-day mortality between the two groups, and segmentectomy is generally regarded as as safe procedure.[25,33,35]

Del Calvo and colleagues[36] performed a retrospective analysis, also using the NCDB, comparing wedge resection to segmentectomy or lobectomy for TC. They found that patients who underwent a wedge resection had worse overall survival at 5 years. Multivariable analysis found that older age, wedge resection, and interestingly use of chemoradiation were all associated with poorer survival.[36] The authors note that individuals who had a segmentectomy or lobectomy were more likely to be upstaged than those who received a wedge resection. Though best practices around adjuvant therapy are not well defined, as discussed above, sufficient lymphadenectomy for staging assists with prognostication. Brown and colleagues[37] conducted a retrospective analysis using the NCDB on the degree of lung resection and lymphadenectomy for cT1aN0M0 carcinoid disease. Although overall survival was not affected by the degree of resection, they found that lymph node upstaging was the strongest predictor of mortality.

## SUMMARY

The rarity of carcinoid tumors has precluded researchers ability to carry out large-scale prospective trials in the same vein as CALGB/ALLIANCE 140503 and COG0802/WJOG4607L. The existing retrospective data on the benefit of anatomic over wedge resection is difficult to parse given the built-in selection bias for patients who are offered wedge resection. It appears that extent of nodal sampling and accurate staging are important long-term prognostic factors. Wedge resections tend to have lower lymph node yields when compared to anatomic resection, casting the latter in a favorable light. Finally, as it may not be possible to differentiate between typical and atypical carcinoid intraoperatively, a more agressive resection strategy should be favored: nodal invasion is an important prognostic factor for AC, and non-anatomic resection may increase disease recurrence.[1] Segmentectomy provides an oncologic resection while preserving as much lung parenchyma as possible, and is a reasonable approach to apply to small, undifferentiated, or known carcinoid lesions. As surgeons become more facile in segmentectomy, it is likely to become the standard approach for carcinoid tumors, with wedge resection and mediastinal lymph node sampling reserved as a second-line approach for marginal surgical candidates.

## CLINICS CARE POINTS

- Bronchopulmonary carcinoid tumors are rare, low-to-intermediate-grade, well-differentiated tumors of neuroendocrine origin.
- Adjuvant or neoadjuvant therapy has limited use only in advanced disease.
- Surgical resection may be curative and is the standard of care for early-stage disease.
- Current consensus guidelines recommend anatomic resection for the treatment of stage I to IIIA disease.

- Though indolent, carcinoids are malignant and should be treated as such.
- Anatomic lung resection, specifically segmentectomy, is a reasonable approach to these tumors.

## DISCLOSURE

The authors have nothing to disclose.

## REFERENCES

1. Caplin ME, Baudin E, Ferolla P, et al. Pulmonary neuroendocrine (carcinoid) tumors: european neuroendocrine tumor society expert consensus and recommendations for best practice for typical and atypical pulmonary carcinoids. Ann Oncol 2015;26(8):1604–20.
2. Yoon JY, Sigel K, Martin J, et al. Evaluation of the prognostic significance of TNM staging guidelines in lung carcinoid tumors. J Thorac Oncol 2019; 14(2):184–92.
3. Travis WD, Brambilla E, Nicholson AG, et al. The 2015 world health organization classification of lung tumors: impact of genetic, clinical and radiologic advances since the 2004 classification. J Thorac Oncol 2015;10(9):1243–60.
4. Bertino EM, Confer PD, Colonna JE, et al. Pulmonary neuroendocrine/carcinoid tumors: a review article. Cancer 2009;115(19):4434–41.
5. Detterbeck FC. Management of carcinoid tumors. Ann Thorac Surg 2010;89(3):998–1005.
6. Sadowski SM, Christ E, Bédat B, et al. Nationwide multicenter study on the management of pulmonary neuroendocrine (carcinoid) tumors. Endocr Connect 2018;7(1):8–15.
7. Stolz A, Harustiak T, Simonek J, et al. Long-term outcomes and prognostic factors of patients with pulmonary carcinoid tumors. Neoplasma 2015;62(3): 478–83.
8. Filosso PL, Rena O, Donati G, et al. Bronchial carcinoid tumors: surgical management and long-term outcome. J Thorac Cardiovasc Surg 2002;123(2): 303–9.
9. Uprety D, Halfdanarson TR, Molina JR, et al. Pulmonary neuroendocrine tumors: adjuvant and systemic treatments. Curr Treat Options Oncol Aug 29 2020; 21(11):86.
10. Baudin E, Caplin M, Garcia-Carbonero R, et al. Lung and thymic carcinoids: ESMO Clinical Practice Guidelines for diagnosis, treatment and follow-up. Ann Oncol 2021;32(4):439–51.
11. Derks JL, Rijnsburger N, Hermans BCM, et al. Clinical-pathologic challenges in the classification of pulmonary neuroendocrine neoplasms and targets on the horizon for future clinical practice. J Thorac Oncol 2021;16(10):1632–46.
12. Nicholson AG, Tsao MS, Beasley MB, et al. The 2021 WHO classification of lung tumors: impact of advances Since 2015. J Thorac Oncol 2022;17(3): 362–87.
13. Metovic J, Barella M, Bianchi F, et al. Morphologic and molecular classification of lung neuroendocrine neoplasms. Virchows Arch 2021;478(1):5–19.
14. Travis WD, Giroux DJ, Chansky K, et al. The IASLC lung cancer staging project: proposals for the inclusion of broncho-pulmonary carcinoid tumors in the forthcoming (seventh) edition of the TNM classification for lung cancer. J Thorac Oncol 2008;3(11): 1213–23.
15. Neuroendocrine and Adrenal Tumors: NCCN Evidence Blocks, Available at: www.nccn.org. Accessed July 19, 2022 2022.
16. Sellke F., del Nido P. and Swanson S., Bronchopulmonary carcinoids. Sabiston & Spencer surgery of the chest, 9th edition, 2016, Elsevier Health Sciences, Philadelphia, PA, chap 22.
17. Gosain R, Groman A, Yendamuri SS, et al. Role of adjuvant chemotherapy in pulmonary carcinoids: an NCDB analysis. Anticancer Res 2019;39(12): 6835–42.
18. Ramirez RA, Thomas K, Jacob A, et al. Adjuvant therapy for lung neuroendocrine neoplasms. World J Clin Oncol 2021;12(8):664–74.
19. Wegner RE, Abel S, Hasan S, et al. The role of adjuvant therapy for atypical bronchopulmonary carcinoids. Lung Cancer 2019;131:90–4.
20. Westin GFM, Alsidawi S, Leventakos K, et al. Impact of adjuvant chemotherapy in non-metastatic node positive bronchial neuroendocrine tumors (BNET). J Clin Oncol 2017;35(15_suppl):8533.
21. Afoke J, Tan C, Hunt I, et al. Is sublobar resection equivalent to lobectomy for surgical management of peripheral carcinoid? Interact Cardiovasc Thorac Surg 2013;16(6):858–63.
22. Walters SL, Canavan ME, Salazar MC, et al. A national study of surgically managed atypical pulmonary carcinoid tumors. Ann Thorac Surg 2021; 112(3):921–7.
23. Machuca TN, Cardoso PF, Camargo SM, et al. Surgical treatment of bronchial carcinoid tumors: a single-center experience. Lung Cancer 2010;70(2):158–62.
24. Rea F, Rizzardi G, Zuin A, et al. Outcome and surgical strategy in bronchial carcinoid tumors: single institution experience with 252 patients. Eur J Cardio Thorac Surg 2007;31(2):186–91.
25. Altorki NK, Wang X, Wigle D, et al. Perioperative mortality and morbidity after sublobar versus lobar resection for early-stage non-small-cell lung cancer: post-hoc analysis of an international, randomised, phase 3 trial (CALGB/Alliance 140503). Lancet Respir Med 2018;6(12):915–24.

26. Suzuki K, Saji H, Aokage K, et al. Comparison of pulmonary segmentectomy and lobectomy: Safety results of a randomized trial. J Thorac Cardiovasc Surg 2019;158(3):895–907.

27. Fox M, Van Berkel V, Bousamra M 2nd, et al. Surgical management of pulmonary carcinoid tumors: sublobar resection versus lobectomy. Am J Surg 2013;205(2):200–8.

28. Yendamuri S, Gold D, Jayaprakash V, et al. Is sublobar resection sufficient for carcinoid tumors? Ann Thorac Surg 2011;92(5):1774–9.

29. Cattoni M, Vallieres E, Brown LM, et al. Sublobar resection in the treatment of peripheral typical carcinoid tumors of the lung. Ann Thorac Surg 2019; 108(3):859–65.

30. Rahouma M, Kamel M, Narula N, et al. Role of wedge resection in bronchial carcinoid (BC tumors: SEER database analysis, J Thor Dis, 11(4), 1355–62.

31. Yan T, Wang K, Liu J, et al. Wedge resection is equal to segmental resection for pulmonary typical carcinoid patients at localized stage: a population-based analysis. PeerJ 2019;7:e7519.

32. Filosso PL, Guerrera F, Falco NR, et al. Anatomical resections are superior to wedge resections for overall survival in patients with Stage 1 typical carcinoids. Eur J Cardio Thorac Surg 2019;55(2):273–9.

33. Bachman KC, Worrell SG, Linden PA, et al. Wedge resection offers similar survival to segmentectomy for typical carcinoid tumors. Semin Thorac Cardiovasc Surg 2022;34(1):293–8.

34. Linden PA, D'Amico TA, Perry Y, et al. Quantifying the safety benefits of wedge resection: a society of thoracic surgery database propensity-matched analysis. Ann Thorac Surg 2014;98(5):1705–12.

35. Handa Y, Tsutani Y, Mimae T, et al. Surgical procedure selection for stage I lung cancer: complex segmentectomy versus wedge resection. Clin Lung Cancer 2021;22(2):e224–33.

36. Del Calvo H, Nguyen DT, Chan EY, et al. Anatomic pulmonary resection is associated with improved survival in typical carcinoid lung tumor patients. J Surg Res 2022;275:352–60.

37. Brown LM, Cooke DT, Jett JR, et al. Extent of resection and lymph node assessment for clinical stage T1aN0M0 typical carcinoid tumors. Ann Thorac Surg 2018;105(1):207–13.

# Sublobar Resections
## Indications and Approaches

Benjamin Wei, MD[a,b,*], Frank Gleason, MD, MSPH[c]

## KEYWORDS

- Non-small cell lung cancer • VATS • Lobectomy • PET-CT • Forced vital capacity

## KEY POINTS

- Improvements in both screening protocols and imaging studies have resulted in an increase in the incidence and prevalence of resectable lung cancer.
- Historically, lobectomy was favored for non-small cell lung cancer but recent evidence indicates sublobar resection, specifically segmentectomy, may have similar oncologic outcomes while maintaining a better postoperative morbidity and lung function profile.
- Sublobar resections can be performed by thoracotomy, video-assisted thoracoscopic surgery, or robotic approach. When determining the operation and approach, patient comorbidities, location of lesion, and anticipated difficulty of operation are critical.

## INTRODUCTION

Sublobar resections are frequently performed operations within thoracic surgery. First described in the 1930s for benign disease, sublobar resections, which include wedge resections and segmentectomy, are now offered for a wide range of benign and malignant diseases.[1] Lung cancer has both high prevalence and cancer-related death rate globally.[2] The implementation of screening protocols and advances in imaging has greatly contributed to the increase in incidence and prevalence of lung cancer worldwide.[3,4] Early oncologic detection has led to a concomitant increase in operative volume because resection is the standard of care for early-stage cancer. Until the 1960s, pneumonectomy was offered for all pulmonary oncologic processes. Lobectomy was introduced and has become the most performed resection for cancer, whereas sublobar resection was reserved for those deemed medically unfit.[4–6] Ongoing debate and investigation is changing practice patterns such that sublobar resections are performed as a safe alternative to lobectomy. With an increasing demand for sublobar resection, an understanding of the anatomy, indications, and perioperative management is critical.

## Anatomy

The right lung is composed of 3 lobes, which are further divided into 10 segments, whereas the left lung is made of 2 lobes, which branch into 8 segments. The right upper lobe has apical, anterior, and posterior segments. The right middle lobe has a lateral and medial segment. The right lower lobe has superior, medial basal, anterior basal, lateral basal, and posterior basal segments. The left upper lobe is made of apicoposterior, lingular, superior, and inferior segments. The left lower lobe comprises the superior, anteromedial basal, lateral basal, and posterior basal segments. Segments are composed of lung parenchyma, typically pyramidal in shape, with a central bronchus, artery, and lymphatic channel. Veins run in the intersegmental planes. This structure allows for resection of a singular unit without disrupting adjacent segments. In contrast to segmentectomy, wedge resection does not require dissection of and ligation of the bronchial, blood, or lymphatic supply to the target lesion.[1,5]

Lung cancer, particularly non-small cell lung cancer (NSCLC), favors lymphatic spread. The typical pulmonary lymphatic drainage flows

a Department of Surgery, Division of Cardiothoracic Surgery, University of Alabama at Birmingham, Birmingham, AL 35233, USA; b Birmingham Veterans Administration Medical Center, Birmingham, AL 35233, USA; c Department of Surgery, University of Alabama at Birmingham, Birmingham, AL 35233, USA
* Corresponding author. 703 19th Street South, Zeigler Research Building, Room 701, Birmingham, AL 35294.
E-mail address: bwei@uab.edu

Thorac Surg Clin 33 (2023) 165–178
https://doi.org/10.1016/j.thorsurg.2023.01.011
1547-4127/23/Published by Elsevier Inc.

through parenchymal vessels toward hilar and mediastinal nodes. Lymphatic channel flow is thought to maintain segmental anatomy unless the mass is in contact with the visceral pleura. Recent study evaluating tumor resections revealed a 66% rate of intersegmental lymphatic drainage in patients with primarily early-stage NSCLC located in the periphery adjacent to visceral pleura.[7]

## Indications

Sublobar resections are indicated for many nonmalignant conditions, including blebs, bullae, infectious causes, pulmonary lacerations from penetrating trauma, and pulmonary lipomas and hamartomas, among other benign lesions.[8] Sublobar resections are also used for metastatic lesions if amenable location-wise because there is no discernible advantage to lobectomy. The role of sublobar resections in primary lung cancer, particularly small ($\leq2$ cm), early-stage NSCLC, is currently under debate. A landmark study by Ginsberg and colleagues randomizing patients with T1N0 peripheral NSCLC found a 30% increase in death rate, 50% increase in death with cancer rate, and 75% increase in recurrence rate for patients undergoing sublobar resection in comparison with lobectomy.[6] Subsequent studies supported lobectomy, showing higher occurrence of positive margins, worse lymph node sampling, and worse disease-free survival in sublobar resection.[9–13] Lymph node resection can be suboptimal in sublobar resection, an important consideration given that intrapulmonary lymph node metastasis can be as high as 22.7% in lesions less than 3 cm.[13] In addition to possible inferior locoregional control and overall survival, segmentectomy is considered technically more challenging than lobectomy.[14] Newer evidence, however, is changing the paradigm for small ($\leq2$ cm), early-stage NSCLC. Multiple studies demonstrate equivalent and even improved survival and cancer-related outcomes for individuals undergoing sublobar resection compared with lobectomy. Additionally, segmentectomy offers lower perioperative morbidity and improved postoperative pulmonary function tests.[10,15–19] The studies supporting and opposing sublobar resection have flaws because most are retrospective in nature with several confounding factors. Recently completed randomized controlled trials comparing sublobar resection and lobectomy for 2 cm or less peripheral NSCLC evaluated the oncologic outcomes as well as impact of resection on respiratory function and hospital length of stay, among other variables.[20] In the study "Segmentectomy versus lobectomy in small-sized peripheral non-small-cell lung cancer (JCOG0802/WJOG4607 L): a multicenter, open-label, phase 3, randomized, controlled, non-inferiority trial," Asamura and colleagues compared outcomes of patients undergoing lobectomy versus segmentectomy. More than 1000 patients undergoing resection for stage IA NSCLC at 70 institutions in Japan from 2009 to 2014 were randomized to either treatment arm. The authors found that those undergoing segmentectomy had a statistically significant 5-year survival benefit (94% vs 91%).[21] These studies validate the preferential use of sublobar resection in primary lung cancer operations, further necessitating the understanding of the approach.

## Wedge Resection

Wedge resection is a nonanatomic removal of a portion of the lung without dissection or ligation of individual vessels or airways. Wedge resection is an option in patients with metastatic lesions. Local recurrence rates are significantly higher for solid tumors undergoing wedge resection with a margin of 5 mm or less for stage 1 NSCLC.[22]

## Segmentectomy

Segmentectomy is a sublobar resection that respects anatomic boundaries. Segmentectomy involves dissection of individual segmental bronchi, arteries, and/or veins, as well as parenchymal transection in the intersegmental planes. This approach provides more accurate oncologic staging due to improved access to hilar lymph nodes and has demonstrated better outcomes compared with wedge resection, radiofrequency ablation, brachytherapy, and radiation therapy.[1,23]

## PREOPERATIVE PLANNING/SURGICAL TREATMENT OPTIONS

Evaluation of patients for sublobar resection begins with obtaining a clinical history and physical examination. Basic laboratory work is sent off next and then high-resolution computed tomography (CT) of the chest is performed. The wide availability of high-quality CT scans has significantly improved the diagnostic ability for clinicians.[11] In evaluating tumors on CT, consolidation tumor ratio of 0.25 or less and large areas of ground glass opacity (GGO) are considered favorable features for consideration of sublobar resection. Those values as well as small size of tumor 2 cm or less suggest increased likelihood of successful sublobar resection.[4,24] Pulmonary function tests are obtained, with focus on forced vital capacity (FVC), forced expiratory volume in 1 second (FEV1), and diffusing capacity of the lung for carbon monoxide (DLCO). Symptomatic patients or those deemed high risk are further evaluated with myocardial stress test and echocardiogram. When cancer is suspected, additional imaging with fusion positron emission tomography-CT scan is obtained to evaluate the primary lesion as well as evaluate for metastatic disease.

The next step in evaluation in evaluating candidacy for sublobar resection is mediastinal staging and obtaining tissue for diagnosis. Mediastinal staging can be performed with mediastinoscopy or endobronchial ultrasound guided fine-needle aspiration biopsy (EBUS-FNA). EBUS is also an excellent approach for obtaining tissue from mediastinal and proximal, large tumors or lymph nodes.[25] Various methods exist for obtaining biopsies of masses and target lymph nodes, ranging from bronchoscopy, fluoroscopic guidance, and electromagnetic navigation bronchoscopy (ENB). Standard bronchoscopes could not go distal to subsegmental bronchi, limiting access to lesions. The advent of virtual and ultrathin bronchoscopes allowed for better diagnostic yield in more peripheral lesions. ENB utilizes 3-dimensional reconstructed CT images and an electromagnetic field generated around the patient's thorax to obtain tissue more accurately for the far periphery by following a virtual pathway to the lesion.[26] The most recent advancement is the coupling of ENB with the robotic platform. Using the virtual map created by the high-resolution CT and electromagnetic field and then Monarch or Ion Endoluminal Platforms, providers can improve diagnostic yield into distal airways previously difficult to access while performing it faster and with minimal complications. Retrospective data shows higher diagnostic yield in smaller, peripheral lesions compared with traditional bronchoscopy in both cadaveric and patient studies.[27,28]

While obtaining tissue for diagnosis, providers can improve the ability of surgeons to identify lesions for sublobar resection by marking them in the same procedure. Some lesions rely on intraoperative palpation to guide resection planes. For deeper/smaller lesions and pure GGOs, however, a preoperative method of localization may be preferred to improve the likelihood of successful resection.[1,5] Options include injecting dye or radiopaque markers. Indocyanine green (ICG) has been proven effective in identifying small lesions for patients subject to sublobar resection.[29] A randomized controlled trial, the Virtual-assisted Lung Mapping (VAL-MAP 2.0), is currently underway to evaluate the utility of combining multispot indocyanine dye marking as well as microcoils, which can be identified with intraoperative fluoroscopy to localize tumors for resection.[30]

## DECIDING BETWEEN SUBLOBAR RESECTION VERSUS LOBECTOMY (PRIMARY LUNG CANCER)

The decision of the type of parenchymal resection to perform is influenced by multiple patient and tumor characteristics. Traditionally, lobectomy has been viewed as the "gold-standard" oncologic operation for NSCLC. However, not all patients are candidates for lobectomy due to pulmonary and nonpulmonary factors. A predicted postoperative DLCO and FEV1 (ppoDLCO and ppoFEV1) of greater than 40% is seen as a minimum threshold for a patient to tolerate lung resection. Therefore, patients with marginal pulmonary function testing may not be viewed as good candidates for lobectomy. Some investigators believe that the minimum threshold for safe lung resection can be lower.[31] Conversely, patients who describe dyspnea, despite acceptable ppoFEV1 and ppoDLCO, can experience worsened symptoms after lobectomy, making sublobar resection a more favorable option. Sublobar resection may also be preferable in patients with small (<2 cm) solid nodules, small solid component of mixed density nodules, and/or pure ground glass opacities, even if appropriate candidacy for lobectomy is established. Outcomes following sublobar resections are comparable to lobectomy in these situations, although the topic remains controversial.[3,4,6,8–17,19,20,24,32] Another consideration favoring a sublobar approach relates to nonpulmonary medical comorbidities that favor a shorter, less complex operation, and/or are believed to significantly limit their overall prognosis and life span. Anatomic considerations may also make the decision between sublobar versus lobar resection obvious. The former may not be possible for centrally located or larger tumors. Traditionally, the presence of hilar or mediastinal lymphadenopathy favored lobectomy over sublobar resection, although recent data suggests the equivalence of these operations for stage III NSCLC.[33] Therefore, provided that these lymph nodes can be sampled, sublobar resection may still be a valid strategy even when nodal disease is suspected and lobectomy is a feasible option.

## DECIDING BETWEEN WEDGE RESECTION VERSUS SEGMENTECTOMY

The decision between wedge resection and segmentectomy for primary lung cancer depends on patient and tumor characteristics. Wedge resection is favored for patients for whom duration of operation and time under general anesthesia is paramount because these typically can be done more quickly. Caution needs to be applied, however, with large lesions or those that are difficult to locate because these characteristics increase the complexity and often the duration of the operation. If a lesion cannot be found, or multiple resections are needed to locate a lesion, the purported time-savings of wedge resection may be negated. In addition, parenchymal transection for larger or deeper wedge resections can be difficult, resulting in bleeding and air leaks that can result in complications that are poorly tolerated. A marginal patient may have a worse outcome with a challenging wedge resection than a more straightforward segmentectomy or lobectomy. The amount of lung removed in a wedge resection compared with segmentectomy can be similar, resulting in similar postoperative pulmonary function and breathing. The conversion rate from a minimally invasive approach to thoracotomy for patients undergoing segmentectomy is higher than that for wedge resection.[34] This should be considered when operating on patients with marginal pulmonary function because a thoracotomy may be poorly tolerated and lead to respiratory complications. Here, a more straightforward wedge resection would provide a better outcome than a segmentectomy that becomes more challenging.

Patients with primary lung cancer who are appropriate surgical candidates and whose tumors are in amenable positions are preferentially offered segmentectomy to wedge resection. Segmentectomy has been shown to yield better margins and locoregional recurrence rates than wedge resection.[16,24] Wedge resection may be favored over segmentectomy for tumors located in between segments in a single lobe, as bisegmentectomy can be technically challenging procedure, especially in the lower lobe. However, a tumor that crosses a fissure and spans segments in 2 different lobes (eg, posterior segment of the right upper lobe and the superior segment of the lower lobe) may be best addressed with bisegmentectomy rather than a wedge resection. Surgeon expertise must also be considered. Segmentectomies can be classified as simple or complex. Simple segmentectomies include superior segmentectomies (segment 6), combined resection of all basilar segments (segments 7–10), left apical trisegmentectomies (segments 1–3), and lingulectomies (segments 4–5). All other individual or combined segmentectomies are considered complex and may require conversion to thoracotomy. Balancing the oncologic benefit

and technical difficulty that may require conversion to thoracotomy in each patient is critical. From a perioperative risk standpoint, a patient may be better off with a wedge resection performed with minimally invasive techniques than a segmentectomy performed via a thoracotomy. The oncologic implications of such a trade-off are not well studied.

For patients with metastatic lesions, wedge resection should generally be considered over segmentectomy, assuming reasonable margins can be achieved. Some lesions, however, may be too deep for wedge resections, in which case segmentectomy can be considered.

## PROCEDURAL APPROACH

We favor perioperative management outlined by the enhanced recovery after lung surgery guidelines by Batchelor and colleagues.[35] In the outpatient setting, this includes emphasis on patient education and smoking cessation. In the perioperative setting, interventions include deep venous thrombosis prophylaxis, antibiotic prophylaxis, strict fluid management, atrial fibrillation prevention with oral low-dose diltiazem, and multimodal pain control.

Patient setup in the operating room is the same regardless of operative approach (ie, thoracotomy, video-assisted thoracoscopic surgery [VATS], or robotic). Patients undergo general anesthesia, and the airway is secured with a double-lumen endotracheal tube. They are then placed in the lateral decubitus position with appropriate padding and the table slightly flexed at the hip. Bronchoscopy is performed to confirm tube position as well as evaluate anatomy.

### Thoracotomy

A serratus-sparing posterior thoracotomy is the preferred open approach. An incision parallel to the ribs is made below the tip of the inferior angle of the scapula. The latissimus dorsi muscle is partially divided, and serratus anterior muscle is mobilized, to expose typically the fifth or sixth intercostal space.

### Video-Assisted Thoracoscopic Surgery

When able, a minimally invasive approach with VATS or robotic assistance is preferred to thoracotomy due to decreased pain, fewer postoperative complications, and shorter hospital stay. For port placement, we typically use a 2-cm camera port in the eighth intercostal space in the midaxillary line and a 3 to 4-cm utility port in the fifth intercostal space in the anterior axillary line. Uniportal

VATS approaches may be used as well; some have found decreased pain when compared with multiport VATS, especially if a subxiphoid location is chosen.[36,37]

## Robotic

Robotic resection is our preferred approach, although there are advantages and disadvantages of robotics compared with VATS. The better visualization and articulating abilities of the robotic instruments allows for a more facile dissection. Using the surgeon's favored approach for anatomic resection (in our case robotic; for others, VATS) should be considered when intraoperative conversion to segmentectomy or lobectomy is significant. Easier hilar and mediastinal lymph node dissection and decreased blood loss may also favor the robotic approach.[38] Intraoperative localization of small and/or deep nodules can be done with same-day percutaneous or navigational marking with ICG using fluorescence imaging that is readily available on robotics platform, whereas specialized VATS cameras with this capability may not be available. Utilization of intraoperative ICG improves visualization of intersegmental planes, allowing for faster sublobar resections with reduced air leak duration and hospital length of stays.[39] ICG use has also been shown to improve oncological margin in sublobar resections in a prospective cohort.[40] VATS, however, allows for palpation of nodules for localization, whereas robotic does not due to the lack of haptic feedback. Instrument palpation through the assistant port is possible but limited due to port location and its size of only 12 to 15 mm in a completely portal technique. Adding or extending an additional port to help with manual palpation or palpation with VATS instruments can be done but is cumbersome. Additionally, assessing the adequacy of a margin during wedge resection can be more challenging with robotics because robotics instruments that "clamp" underneath the nodule to help ensure an adequate margin are not available at the present time. The selection of robotics versus VATS for a sublobar resection depends on surgeon experience, relative likelihood of wedge resection versus segmentectomy, possible need for conversion to lobectomy, need for intraoperative localization, size of targeted nodule, and logistical factors.

Typical port placement for a robotic segmentectomy is shown in **Fig. 1**. The camera is located either in the seventh or eighth intercostal space, based on the operative target being in the upper (seventh) or middle/lower (eighth) lobe. Ports are spaced so that the posterior robotic arm (port 3),

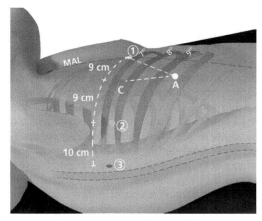

**Fig. 1.** Port positioning for robotic sublobar resection. (*From* Wei B, Cerfolio RJ. Robotic lobectomy: Left Upper Lobectomy. Operative Techniques in Thoracic and Cardiovascular Surgery. 2016;21(3):230-248.)

used for retraction, is located 4 cm lateral from the spinous process. Each additional arm is spaced 9 cm apart to avoid collisions. The assistant port (A) is triangulated behind the camera port and the most anterior port. For wedge resections, parenchymal transection more commonly is performed with a hand-held stapler via the assistant port. For segmentectomies, the distance from the port to the target anatomy should be considered when robotic stapling is anticipated. The right and left arms of the robot should be positioned far enough away from the structures to be stapled to ensure their angle of approach is not overly steep. Therefore, ports 1 and 2 (see **Fig. 1**) may be staggered to a lower interspace than the camera port.

## Lymph Node Dissection

Removal of mediastinal lymph nodes is the first step of sublobar resection. We proceed from inferior to superior and go around the hilum during this process. On the right side, we divide the inferior ligament, and then obtain lymph nodes from stations 9, 8, 7, 4R, and 2R. On the left side, we perform lymph node dissection from stations 9, 8, 7, 6, and 5 from their respective locations. Lymph nodes may be taken from the 4L station through the left chest as well. Hilar lymph nodes at levels 10 and 11 may be taken during the process as they are seen during retraction and dividing the mediastinal pleura to "lengthen the hilum." Nodal dissection is performed first because this exposes important vascular and bronchial structures while allowing time for the evaluation of lymph nodes with frozen section to determine if metastatic disease is present.[1,41]

## Wedge Resection

Wedge resections are often less technically demanding and require less operative time than segmentectomy. They can often be performed with a minimally invasive approach, frequently relying on palpation to guide resection. A distance of 5 mm or greater from the pleural surface for nodules 1 cm or less in diameter, depth-to-size ratio of the nodule of less than 1, pure ground-glass opacities, and mixed density lesions with a small solid component may be nearly impossible to palpate.[42,43] This can necessitate a thoracotomy to allow for palpation of smaller lesions. Localization methods exist including injection of dye, hook-wires, or coils by a percutaneous or guided broncho-scopic approach. An alternative strategy for nodules unable to be palpated is resecting the general area based on nodule location inferred from the CT scan. Conversely, larger and deeper lesions may be difficult or even impossible to safely perform wedge resections for. Grasping the edge of the lung and including it in the parenchyma to be removed, even if the nodule is located a bit farther from the edge itself, may help with obtaining a larger margin, although at the cost of additional lung tissue lost. Nodules located in the fissure may require further dissection or even division of the fissure in order to expose enough parenchyma for stapling beneath the lesion. Particular care should be noted when performing wedge resections on nodules located centrally on the concave surfaces of the lung, such as the lung base, because retraction of this area to achieve an adequate margin can be challenging. Staplers with a taller height may need to be used for deep wedges or thicker lung tissue. Vascular structures of the lung are generally safe during wedge resection, although troublesome bleeding can be encountered from subsegmental and even segmental branches on deep wedge resections. Careful preoperative planning is necessary to allow triangulation with ports and lesion location. When not resecting anatomic boundaries, lung tissue can shift in the stapler affecting margins obtained. Sato and colleagues recommend utilizing the incomplete tissue-grasping technique to improve accuracy. The stapler is gently set alongside the lesion while forceps pull the desired lung parenchyma into the partially opened stapler.[29] Margins are critical in oncologic resections because local recurrence rate can double if margins of less than 1 cm are obtained compared to 1 cm or greater.[32] In addition, hilar nodal dissection performed during wedge resections is generally inferior, as segmental structures are not dissected and therefore lymph nodes in these locations are not typically sampled or removed.

## Segmentectomy

Each segmentectomy requires identification and dissection of the supplying bronchus, artery, and/or vein. A "true" segmentectomy requires division of at least 2 of the abovementioned structures. Staplers are typically used for division of structures, although sutures, clips, and energy devices can be used on vessels. Given that the bronchus is centrally located, the blood supplying vessels generally need to be transected before fully exposing the bronchus. Care must be taken with venous ligation because adjacent segmental venous drainage may come into the field. Vessel loops or ties are used to provide retraction for better visualization to improve safety of dividing structures. Intersegmental planes are divided with energy devices or staplers, depending on surgeon experience.[1,41] Intraoperative bronchoscopy, selective ventilation, and ICG can help delineate segmental boundaries.[1] Preoperative CT scans are helpful to decide on the anatomic appropriateness of segmentectomy. Software can be used to assist in this analysis.[25,26] Intraoperative findings, however, may dictate conversion to either a wedge resection or lobectomy.

First, the vein draining the segment(s) to be resected is identified. For simple segmentectomy, this is generally a straightforward process because the vein to be preserved is identified and the vein to be divided is transected. For complex segmentectomy, the identification of the relevant vein can be more difficult, especially for individual basilar segmentectomies. If the identity of the vein to be ligated is in doubt, the portion of lung to be resected can be grasped, and the vein under the greatest tension is selected for ligation. The ligated vein also tends to be the one with the most direct trajectory between the central hilum and the target segment. It is important to ligate the correct vein because the location of the cut stump will direct the division of future structures. Division of the vein is followed by distal dissection of the segment, which exposes the segmental artery and bronchus. This dissection may require cautery division of parenchyma. There is often more tightly adherent lung parenchyma that needs to be dissected off segmental structures in comparison to lobar structures. When a complete fissure is encountered, the ligation of the segmental artery can either be performed before the vein from the fissure rather than in the "same direction" as the vein was approached.[44] Often both the artery and vein need to be divided before a clear view and approach to the segmental bronchus can be obtained. The angles to safely ligate segmental structures can be difficult to achieve and therefore planning on being able to staple from both the "left" and "right" robotic arms, and even potentially via the assistant port, can be helpful. Once the hilar structures are divided, parenchymal transection is performed. The injection of 10 mg of ICG intravenously can help demarcate the boundaries of the segment, which are then quickly marked with electrocautery before the dye has a chance to diffuse (**Fig. 2**). It is critical to ensure that the divided hilar structures are located in the specimen during this process. Preconditioning of the line of transection by compressing it with a hand-held instrument or even preclosing of the stapler and walking it along the line of transection may be helpful to deal with what is often a thick area of lung.

## TECHNICAL DETAILS OF INDIVIDUAL SEGMENTECTOMIES

The major steps of the more commonly performed simple and complex individual segmentectomies with a robotic technique follows. Individual segmentectomies in the right middle lobe and lingula are rarely performed and not discussed further.[45] A standard mediastinal lymph node dissection and opening up the mediastinal pleura to lengthen the hilum is performed before starting to ligate hilar structures. After division of the relevant hilar structures, the boundary of the segment can be demarcated with 10 mg of intravenous ICG dye or ventilation of the operative lung and then divided with the stapler. At times, transection of the parenchyma earlier in the operation can be helpful to facilitate encircling and division of the hilar structures. Division of *either* the arterial supply or venous drainage of the segment permits the use of ICG to demarcate the parenchyma. Details of a robotic approach are provided but the order of

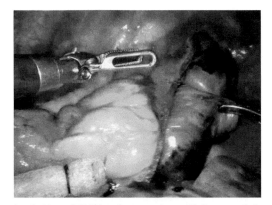

**Fig. 2.** Use of ICG for demarcation of left upper lobe apicoposterior segment before parenchymal transection (wedge resection performed previously).

division and concepts discussed can be applied to VATS or open segmentectomy. We prefer a vein-first approach for hypothetical oncologic benefits of less shedding of tumor cells into the circulation.[46]

### Right Upper Lobe Posterior Segmentectomy

- Retract right upper lobe superiorly and anteriorly.
- Dissect level 11 lymph node between right upper lobe and bronchus intermedius
- Open major fissure posteriorly to visualize the posterior segmental vein. This may be approached by stapling just the posterior aspect of the fissure alone. Alternatively, a subadventitial plane can be developed along the course of the ongoing pulmonary artery in the fissure and the entire fissure can be transected from anterior to posterior with staplers, although this increases the surface area of stapled lung with the resultant increased potential for air leak.
- Divide posterior segmental vein, which typically reveals the posterior segmental artery.
- Dissect and divide the posterior segmental artery.
- Visualize and divide posterior segmental bronchus.

### Right Upper Lobe Apical Segmentectomy

- Retract right upper lobe posteriorly to view the anterior hilum.
- Locate, dissect, and divide the apical vein, the most cephalad branch of the upper lobe veins.
- Expose and ligate the apical artery with a stapler directed from anterior to posterior in a near horizontal fashion. A truncus artery that supplies both the apical and anterior segments needs to be traced distally until the bifurcation is reached and just the apical segmental artery is divided.
- Dissect the distal apical bronchus, which can be quite deep in the hilum. This may require anterior lung retraction to take a posterior approach.

### Right Upper Lobe Anterior Segment

- Retract right upper lobe posteriorly to view the anterior hilum.
- Identify and divide the anterior vein, the second most cephalad branch of the right upper lobe vein.
- Dissect hilum distally and inferiorly toward the uncut posterior segmental vein running underneath the right upper lobe toward the fissure.

This reveals the anterior segmental artery, which can be isolated and divided. This may require a nearly vertical angle of the stapler that travels from the feet to the head of the patient. Alternatively, a truncus artery that supplies both the apical and anterior segments needs to be dissected distally until the bifurcation is reached and just the anterior segmental artery is divided.

- Dissect and divide the anterior bronchus, potentially with a near-vertical stapler alignment.
- Dividing the anterior aspect of the horizontal fissure early with the right robotic arm can help to achieve the necessary angles for division of hilar structures in right upper lobe anterior segmentectomy, which then can be taken more easily from the left robotic arm to avoid injury to the apical vessels.

### Superior Segmentectomy (Right or Left)

- Retract the lung anteriorly to establish a posterior view.
- Identify the superior segmental vein, the most cephalad branch of the lower lobe vein, then isolate and divide.
- If there is a complete fissure, dissect the superior segmental artery and divide with a near horizontal pass of the stapler from right to left (right lung) or left to right (left lung).
- If there is an incomplete fissure, approach and divide the superior segmental bronchus from a posterior view. Removing the level 12 lymph node between the superior segmental bronchus and ongoing lower lobe bronchus before approaching the bronchus can be beneficial. Care should be taken to define the distance and dissect open the space between the superior segmental bronchus and superior segmental artery when passing the stapler. Alternatively, the posterior aspect of the fissure can be divided to expose the superior segmental artery and the artery divided before the bronchus.
- Dissect and divide the remaining hilar structure (artery or bronchus)

### Basilar Segmentectomy (Right or Left)

- Basilar segmentectomies can be the most challenging segmentectomies to perform due to more difficult identification of the target vessels. Division of the correct initial vessel, typically vein, is extremely important because this will dictate the identification and division of additional structures.

- Identify the superior segmental vein first; then dissect the basilar veins distally to visualize their origin.
- Grasp the target segment then divide the segmental vein under the most tension (**Fig. 3**).[44]
- Dissect the segmental bronchus distally to confirm its common origin with the vein, then isolate and divide (**Fig. 4**).
- For anterior basilar segmentectomies especially, approaching the artery to the basilar segments through a complete fissure, or after transection of a partial fissure, can facilitate identification and division of the segmental artery before division of the segmental bronchus.
- Dissect and divide the remaining hilar structures.

### Left Upper Lobe Apical Trisegmentectomy (Lingula Sparing Lobectomy)

- Retract the lung posteriorly for an anterior view.
- Identify and preserve the lingular vein.
- Identify the cephalad branch of the upper lobe vein as the upper division vein and then divide.
- Expose and divide the arteries to the apical trisegment. The order in which this is done can vary. If there is a complete or near-complete fissure, which is typically the case for the left lung, it can be easier to approach the posterior artery first with the lung-retracted anterosuperior. Then the apical and anterior arteries can be divided from either a posterior or an anterior approach, depending on which angles are more favorable for the stapler. At times, dividing the upper division bronchus first may help facilitate the approach to certain segmental arteries.

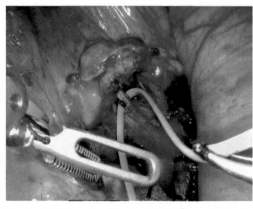

**Fig. 3.** Basilar vein dissected distally and tension applied to identify vein to be divided.

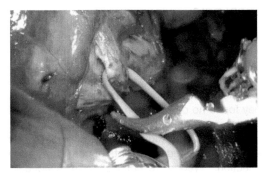

Fig. 4. Preparation for division of anterior segmental bronchus to right lower lobe.

- Follow the upper lobe bronchus to its bifurcation, then isolate and staple the upper division bronchus.

### Left Upper Lobe Posterior/Apicoposterior Segmentectomy

- If performing an apicoposterior bisegmentectomy, retract the lung posteriorly, and isolate/divide the most cranial segmental vein, which drains the apicoposterior segments.
- For an isolated left upper lobe posterior segmentectomy, the artery is typically divided first because the vein is not easily identifiable, and its specific division can be omitted. Resection of the apical segment of the left upper lobe alone is quite challenging but if attempted, it can be performed with a similar approach to right upper lobe apical segmentectomy.
- Retract the lung superiorly and anteriorly.
- Isolate/divide the posterior segmental artery located in the posterior fissure, dividing the fissure if needed.
- If appropriate, isolate and divide the apical segmental artery, exposing the bronchus to the apicoposterior segment.
- Dissect and divide the posterior, or both the apical/posterior bronchi, with the left robotic arm (**Fig. 5**).

### Left Upper Lobe Anterior Segmentectomy

- Retract the lung posteriorly.
- Identify and preserve the lingular vein.
- Isolate and divide the anterior segmental vein, usually with the right robotic arm. It can be difficult to determine the anterior versus apical vein but the anterior vein(s) is more caudal.
- Isolate/divide the anterior segmental artery or bronchus based on the optimal angle/accessibility.
- Divide the final segmental hilar structure.

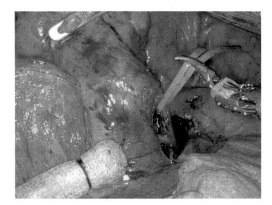

Fig. 5. Preparation for division of left upper lobe posterior segmental bronchus.

### Lingulectomy

- Retract the lung posteriorly.
- Identify the left superior and inferior pulmonary veins.
- Divide the lingular vein, the more inferior/caudal branch of the bifurcating left superior pulmonary vein, usually with the right robotic arm.
- Identify and divide the 1 or 2 lingular arteries in the fissure, usually with the left robotic arm.
- Lingular arteries are approached next because the lingular bronchus is surrounded by lung parenchyma/hilar structures and not easily accessible yet. Typically, 1 or 2 lingular arteries are identified in the fissure, and divided.
- Dissect the left upper lobe bronchus distally to its bifurcation. Divide the lingular bronchus, which is the more caudal of the structures running to the same area as the divided arteries and vein. This is typically performed with the left robotic arm.

### Recovery and Rehabilitation

We utilize many of the perioperative interventions from the enhanced recovery after lung surgery guidelines.[35] Chest tubes are transitioned to water seal early and removed once output less than 500 mL/d and no air leak is visible, often on postoperative day one. Early patient mobilization and aggressive pulmonary physiotherapy are also important. The use of multimodal pain regimens allows for adequate pain control while minimizing opioid use.

### Outcomes

#### Perioperative
Patients who undergo segmentectomy have similar complication profiles as those who undergo

lobectomy.[18] The overall 30-day mortality ranges from 0.9% to 3%. Morbidity ranges from 15% to 39%, the most common complications being pneumonia, hypoxia, atrial fibrillation, prolonged air leak, and bleeding.[1] Patients undergoing wedge resection seem to have a significantly lower complication rate compared with those undergoing lobectomy.[47] Segmentectomy has been associated with a better quality of life and dyspnea compared with lobectomy at 12 months after surgery.[48]

## PULMONARY FUNCTION

Sublobar resections are reported to have an impact on postoperative FEV1 and DLCO but patients are expected to maintain 90% of preoperative function.[5] Sublobar resections lead to greater preservation of lung function than lobectomy. Multiple studies have demonstrated the overall advantages of segmentectomy versus lobectomy with regards to lung function.[49,50] However, differences in lung function may take time to manifest. Saito and colleagues found that the advantages in pulmonary function for patients undergoing *open* segmentectomy compared with lobectomy were significant at 6 months, but not 1 month, following surgery.[51] Complex and simple segmentectomy have shown to demonstrate similar preservation of lung function.[52] The number of segments being removed can affect the purported benefits of sublobar resection over lobectomy. For instance, Nomori and colleagues demonstrated that the percentage of preoperative lung function preserved was 95% for single segmentectomy, compared with 86% for lobectomy.[53] This same study, however, demonstrated no significant difference in the loss of pulmonary function between lobectomy and resection of 2 or more segments of lung. The actual loss of lung function tends to be more than expected for segmentectomy and less than expected for lobectomy.[54,55] In the study by Chen and colleagues, removing more than 50% of the segments in a given lobe negated any significant mitigation in the loss of FEV1, FVC, or DLCO compared with the corresponding lobectomy. Therefore, certain segmentectomies may not be worth the additional technical complexity (eg, resecting 2 segments in the right upper lobe, or resecting all of the basilar segments but preserving the superior segment in a lower lobectomy). Although some think that using electrocautery rather than stapling in segmental resection may lead to less distortion of the parenchyma and improved lung function, this is not widely supported by the data, and does carry a higher risk of postoperative air leak.[56]

## ONCOLOGIC

Using data from the National Lung Screening Trial Database, Kamel and colleagues compared outcomes of sublobar resection to lobectomy for patients with stage I NSCLC with a propensity match analysis. In comparing 127 patients in each arm, they found no difference in 5-year overall survival or cancer-specific survival between the 2 groups. The caveat of this study is that the sublobar group primarily consisted of patients undergoing wedge resection. Wedge resections have historically been considered a lesser oncologic operation in comparison to lobectomy given the nonanatomical nature of the margins as well as inferior yield of lymph nodes. This stance is supported by a study by Salazar and colleagues who, using SEER Medicare data, showed higher risk of mortality (HR 1.68, 95% CI [1.52–1.86]) in patients with 2 cm or less NSCLC undergoing wedge resection in comparison to lobectomy with a comorbidity-related life expectancy of more than 5 years.[57] Conversely, patients with a comorbidity-related life expectancy of less than 5 years who underwent lobectomy had more than double the 90-day mortality rate (9% vs 4%) than those undergoing wedge resection. This shows that each operative approach has utility in the appropriate patient setting. Cao and colleagues compared lobectomy, segmentectomy, and wedge resection for stage IA NSCLC using SEER Medicare data in terms of lung cancer-specific survival.[58] They found for lesions of 2 to 3 cm, lobectomy offered the best outcomes, whereas there was no difference for lesions less than 1 cm among the operations performed. Often, wedge is presented as being reserved for patients who are not candidates for lobectomy for various reasons, including age. Mimae and colleagues compared outcomes for 892 patients aged 80 years or older with 2 cm or less NSCLC.[59] They found the 3-year overall survival did not differ between patients offered wedge resection compared with lobectomy. An additional regression analysis did not find the procedure offered as being a predictor of death in this patient population. Dolan and colleagues performed a retrospective propensity-matched analysis of patients at their institution and identified that those undergoing wedge resection had significantly lower postoperative complication rates compared with those undergoing lobectomy (19% vs 34%), while maintaining equivalent overall and disease-free survival.[47] Among this group, patients undergoing wedge resection had worse locoregional recurrence-free survival rates compared with patients undergoing lobectomy but this difference was eliminated if margins of more than 1 cm were obtained.

A growing amount of evidence is accumulating that legitimizes segmentectomy as an oncologic operation when compared with lobectomy. Chan and colleagues performed a retrospective study at their institution during a 13-year period comparing outcomes of patients with T1c NSCLC undergoing segmentectomy versus lobectomy.[60] Utilizing a propensity match, there was no difference found in postoperative complications, disease recurrence, or 5-year survival. Another single institution, retrospective study was performed by Dolan and colleagues during an 18-year period for patients with stage I NSCLC undergoing lobectomy versus superior segmentectomy and found equivalent 5-year overall survival, disease-free survival, and locoregional-recurrence-free survival.[61] One limitation to sublobar resection is a lower yield of lymph nodes. This was confirmed by a 16-year retrospective analysis by Kamel and colleagues for patients at their institution with stage IA adenocarcinoma.[62] Patients who underwent lobectomy had a median lymph node yield of 14, compared with 7 for segmentectomy ($P < .01$). This resulted in a higher rate of nodal upstaging for those undergoing lobectomy. Despite this, there was no statistical difference in 5-year recurrence-free survival or 5-year cancer-specific survival. This calls to question the advantage of the nodal yield in lobectomy if outcomes may not truly be impacted. Razi and colleagues further investigated outcomes for patients with pathologic N1 and N2 disease who underwent lobectomy compared with segmentectomy.[63] They found that adjuvant chemotherapy, not the operation performed, had an impact on survival for these individuals. Onaitis and colleagues compared outcomes of patients with stage I NSCLC undergoing lobectomy to those undergoing segmentectomy using the STS database linked with Medicare data and found no statistical difference in survival. Another study by Bao and colleagues confirms the finding of equivalence for cancer-specific survival for patients undergoing segmentectomy compared with lobectomy for 2 cm or less NSCLC.[64] They also showed that patients with lesions larger than this should undergo lobectomy because it offers a better cancer-specific survival. A noninferiority randomized controlled trial comparing 1106 patients undergoing lobectomy versus segmentectomy for stage IA NSCLC at 70 different institutions in Japan found better 5-year survival (94% vs 91%), although the rate of local relapse favors lobectomy (5.4% vs 10.5%).[21] Contrary to the previously mentioned studies showing equivalent outcomes, Baig and colleagues queried the National Cancer Database for patients with 2 cm or less NSCLC undergoing resection and found a statistically significant difference in survival favoring lobectomy to segmentectomy (88 vs 68 months).[65] Given the variety of outcomes reported and retrospective nature of these studies, a true consensus reliant on high-level evidence has not been attained with respect to the equivalence of segmentectomy to lobectomy. A recent publication by Saji and colleagues provides the highest level of evidence to date. They performed a randomized controlled, noninferiority trial at 70 institutions in Japan for patients with 2 cm or less NSCLC with consolidation to tumor ratio greater than 0.5.[21] Patients were randomly assigned to lobectomy or segmentectomy arms. They found similar 5-year relapse-free survival rates and no 30 or 90-day mortalities. Interestingly, the lung sparing segmentectomy did not provide clinically significant benefits to postoperative FEV1 and had almost double the rates of local recurrence (10.5% vs 5.4%, $P = .0018$). Despite this, the overall survival was actually *better* in the segmentectomy cohort. This study is the highest level of evidence available in the comparison of segmentectomy to lobectomy for small NSCLC and supports the sublobar approach as a reasonable alternative to lobectomy in a selected population.

## SUMMARY

- Improvements in both screening protocols and imaging studies have resulted in an increase in the incidence and prevalence of resectable lung cancer.
- The right lung consists of 3 lobes, which are further divided into 10 segments, whereas the left lung is made of 2 lobes, which branch into 8 segments.
- Nonmalignant conditions warranting sublobar resection include blebs, bullae, infection, and laceration.
- Sublobar resection may offer improved morbidity and preserved lung function compared with lobectomy.
- Wedge resection can be quick and better tolerated by some patients.
- Segmentectomy involves identifying and dividing the bronchus and vasculature supply.
- Sublobar resections can be performed by thoracotomy, VATS, or robotic approach.
- When determining the operation and approach, patient comorbidities, location of lesion, and anticipated difficulty of operation are critical.
- Lobectomy has long been considered the gold standard for oncologic resections but

there is an ongoing debate on the role of sublobar resection for small, early-stage NSCLC with a recently published randomized controlled trial favoring segmentectomy.

## CLINICS CARE POINTS

- Nonmalignant conditions warranting sublobar resection include blebs, bullae, infection, and laceration.
- Lobectomy has long been considered the gold standard for oncologic resections but there is an ongoing debate on the role of sublobar resection for small, early-stage NSCLC with a recently published RCT favoring segmentectomy.
- Wedge resection can be quick and better tolerated by some patients but those with larger tumors in locations that are more challenging to approach may benefit from lobectomy.
- Segmentectomy involves identifying and dividing the bronchus and vasculature supply. The vein-first approach may result in less shedding of tumor cells into the circulation.
- The robotic approach offers better visualization, instrument articulation, easier hilar and mediastinal nodal dissection, and decreased blood loss, whereas VATS is less expensive than robotic approach and allows palpation of nodes.

## DISCLOSURES

The authors have nothing to disclose with regard to commercial support.

## REFERENCES

1. Sugarbaker DJ. Sugarbaker's adult chest surgery. Third edition. New York: McGraw Hill Education; 2020.
2. Hoy H, Lynch T, Beck M. Surgical Treatment of Lung Cancer. Crit Care Nurs Clin 2019;31(3):303–13.
3. Yaldız D, Yakut FC, Kaya Ş Örs, et al. The Role of Sublobar Resection in T1 N0 Non-Small-Cell Pulmonary Carcinoma. Turk Thorac J 2020;21(5):308–13.
4. Suzuki K, Watanabe SI, Wakabayashi M, et al. A single-arm study of sublobar resection for ground-glass opacity dominant peripheral lung cancer. J Thorac Cardiovasc Surg 2022;163(1):289–301.e282.
5. Mathisen DJ, Morse CR. Thoracic surgery. Lung resections, bronchoplasty. Philadelphia: Wolters Kluwer; 2015.
6. Ginsberg RJ, Rubinstein LV. Randomized trial of lobectomy versus limited resection for T1 N0 non-small cell lung cancer. Lung Cancer Study Group. Ann Thorac Surg 1995;60(3):615–22. ; discussion 622-613.
7. Fourdrain A, Epailly J, Blanchard C, et al. Lymphatic drainage of lung cancer follows an intersegmental pathway within the visceral pleura. Lung Cancer 2021;154:118–23.
8. Şahin M, Yenigün MB, Kocaman G, et al. Sublobar resections in early-stage non-small cell lung cancer. Turk Gogus Kalp Damar Cerrahisi Derg 2019;27(3):367–73.
9. Cao C, Tian DH, Fu B, et al. The problem with sublobar resections. J Thorac Dis 2018;10(Suppl 26):S3224–6.
10. Cao C, Gupta S, Chandrakumar D, et al. Meta-analysis of intentional sublobar resections versus lobectomy for early stage non-small cell lung cancer. Ann Cardiothorac Surg 2014;3(2):134–41.
11. Berfield KS, Wood DE. Sublobar resection for stage IA non-small cell lung cancer. J Thorac Dis 2017;9(Suppl 3):S208–10.
12. Whitson BA, Groth SS, Andrade RS, et al. Survival after lobectomy versus segmentectomy for stage I non-small cell lung cancer: a population-based analysis. Ann Thorac Surg 2011;92(6):1943–50.
13. Deng HY, Tang X, Zhou Q. Sublobar resection: an alternative to lobectomy in treating stage I non-small-cell lung cancer? Eur J Cardio Thorac Surg 2020;57(3):613.
14. Gossot D. Lobar or sublobar resection for early-stage lung cancer: at the crossroads. Eur J Cardio Thorac Surg 2021;60(6):1295–6.
15. Altorki NK, Wang X, Wigle D, et al. Perioperative mortality and morbidity after sublobar versus lobar resection for early-stage non-small-cell lung cancer: post-hoc analysis of an international, randomised, phase 3 trial (CALGB/Alliance 140503). Lancet Respir Med 2018;6(12):915–24.
16. Sihoe ADL. Should sublobar resection be offered for screening-detected lung nodules? Transl Lung Cancer Res 2021;10(5):2418–26.
17. Yendamuri S, Sharma R, Demmy M, et al. Temporal trends in outcomes following sublobar and lobar resections for small ($\leq$ 2 cm) non-small cell lung cancers–a Surveillance Epidemiology End Results database analysis. J Surg Res 2013;183(1):27–32.
18. Huang CS, Hsu PK, Chen CK, et al. Surgeons' preference sublobar resection for stage I NSCLC less than 3 cm. Thorac Cancer 2020;11(4):907–17.
19. Kamel MK, Lee B, Harrison SW, et al. Sublobar resection is comparable to lobectomy for screen-detected lung cancer. J Thorac Cardiovasc Surg 2022;163(6):1907–15.
20. Nakamura K, Saji H, Nakajima R, et al. A phase III randomized trial of lobectomy versus limited

resection for small-sized peripheral non-small cell lung cancer (JCOG0802/WJOG4607L). Jpn J Clin Oncol 2010;40(3):271–4.

21. Saji H, Okada M, Tsuboi M, et al. Segmentectomy versus lobectomy in small-sized peripheral non-small-cell lung cancer (JCOG0802/WJOG4607L): a multicentre, open-label, phase 3, randomised, controlled, non-inferiority trial. Lancet 2022; 399(10335):1607–17.

22. Moon Y, Lee KY, Moon SW, et al. Sublobar Resection Margin Width Does Not Affect Recurrence of Clinical N0 Non-small Cell Lung Cancer Presenting as GGO-Predominant Nodule of 3 cm or Less. World J Surg 2017;41(2):472–9.

23. Chen E, Wang J, Jia C, et al. Sublobar resection with intraoperative brachytherapy versus sublobar resection alone for early-stage non-small-cell lung cancer: a meta-analysis. Interact Cardiovasc Thorac Surg 2021;33(3):377–84.

24. Sakurai H, Asamura H. Sublobar resection for early-stage lung cancer. Transl Lung Cancer Res 2014; 3(3):164–72.

25. Jiang J, Chang SH, Kent AJ, et al. Current Novel Advances in Bronchoscopy. Front Surg 2020;7:596925.

26. Simoff MJ, Pritchett MA, Reisenauer JS, et al. Shape-sensing robotic-assisted bronchoscopy for pulmonary nodules: initial multicenter experience using the Ion™ Endoluminal System. BMC Pulm Med 2021;21(1):322.

27. Kumar A, Caceres JD, Vaithilingam S, et al. Robotic Bronchoscopy for Peripheral Pulmonary Lesion Biopsy: Evidence-Based Review of the Two Platforms. Diagnostics 2021;11(8).

28. Agrawal A, Hogarth DK, Murgu S. Robotic bronchoscopy for pulmonary lesions: a review of existing technologies and clinical data. J Thorac Dis 2020; 12(6):3279–86.

29. Sato M. Strategies to improve the accuracy of lung stapling in uniportal and multiportal thoracoscopic sublobar lung resections. Eur J Cardio Thorac Surg 2020;58(Suppl_1):i108–10.

30. Zhang C, Lin H, Fu R, et al. Application of indocyanine green fluorescence for precision sublobar resection. Thorac Cancer 2019;10(4):624–30.

31. Brunelli A, Refai M, Salati M, et al. Predicted versus observed FEV1 and DLCO after major lung resection: a prospective evaluation at different postoperative periods. Ann Thorac Surg 2007;83(3):1134–9.

32. El-Sherif A, Fernando HC, Santos R, et al. Margin and local recurrence after sublobar resection of non-small cell lung cancer. Ann Surg Oncol 2007; 14(8):2400–5.

33. Mynard N, Nasar A, Rahouma M, et al. Extent of resection influences survival in early-stage lung cancer with occult nodal disease. Ann Thorac Surg 2022;114(3):959–67.

34. Tong C, Li T, Huang C, et al. Risk Factors and Impact of Conversion to Thoracotomy From 20,565 Cases of Thoracoscopic Lung Surgery. Ann Thorac Surg 2020;109(5):1522–9.

35. Batchelor TJP, Rasburn NJ, Abdelnour-Berchtold E, et al. Guidelines for enhanced recovery after lung surgery: recommendations of the Enhanced Recovery After Surgery (ERAS®) Society and the European Society of Thoracic Surgeons (ESTS). Eur J Cardio Thorac Surg 2019;55(1):91–115.

36. Chen J, Volpi S, Ali JM, et al. Comparison of postoperative pain and quality of life between uniportal subxiphoid and intercostal video-assisted thoracoscopic lobectomy. J Thorac Dis 2020;12(7): 3582–90.

37. Yang X, Wang L, Zhang C, et al. The Feasibility and Advantages of Subxiphoid Uniportal Video-Assisted Thoracoscopic Surgery in Pulmonary Lobectomy. World J Surg 2019;43(7):1841–9.

38. Yang HX, Woo KM, Sima CS, et al. Long-term Survival Based on the Surgical Approach to Lobectomy For Clinical Stage I Nonsmall Cell Lung Cancer: Comparison of Robotic, Video-assisted Thoracic Surgery, and Thoracotomy Lobectomy. Ann Surg 2017;265(2):431–7.

39. Ng CS, Ong BH, Chao YK, et al. Use of indocyanine green fluorescence imaging in thoracic and esophageal surgery. Ann Thorac Surg 2022.

40. Mehta M, Patel YS, Yasufuku K, et al. Near-infrared mapping with indocyanine green is associated with an increase in oncological margin length in minimally invasive segmentectomy. J Thorac Cardiovasc Surg 2019;157(5):2029–35.

41. Wei B, Cerfolio R. Technique of robotic segmentectomy. J Vis Surg 2017;3:140.

42. Suzuki K, Nagai K, Yoshida J, et al. Video-assisted thoracoscopic surgery for small indeterminate pulmonary nodules: indications for preoperative marking. Chest 1999;115(2):563–8.

43. Imperatori A, Nardecchia E, Cattoni M, et al. Perioperative identifications of non-palpable pulmonary nodules: a narrative review. J Thorac Dis 2021; 13(4):2524–31.

44. Liu C, Liao H, Guo C, et al. Single-direction thoracoscopic basal segmentectomy. J Thorac Cardiovasc Surg 2020;160(6):1586–94.

45. Handa Y, Tsutani Y, Mimae T, et al. Complex Segmentectomy for Hypermetabolic Clinical Stage IA Non-Small Cell Lung Cancer. Ann Thorac Surg 2022;113(4):1317–24.

46. Wei S, Guo C, He J, et al. Effect of Vein-First vs Artery-First Surgical Technique on Circulating Tumor Cells and Survival in Patients With Non-Small Cell Lung Cancer: A Randomized Clinical Trial and Registry-Based Propensity Score Matching Analysis. JAMA Surg 2019;154(7):e190972.

47. Dolan D, Swanson SJ, Gill R, et al. Survival and Recurrence Following Wedge Resection Versus Lobectomy for Early-Stage Non-Small Cell Lung Cancer. Semin Thorac Cardiovasc Surg 2022;34(2): 712–23.

48. Stamatis G, Leschber G, Schwarz B, et al. Perioperative course and quality of life in a prospective randomized multicenter phase III trial, comparing standard lobectomy versus anatomical segmentectomy in patients with non-small cell lung cancer up to 2 cm, stage IA (7th edition of TNM staging system). Lung Cancer 2019;138:19–26.

49. Wang X, Guo H, Hu Q, et al. Pulmonary function after segmentectomy versus lobectomy in patients with early-stage non-small-cell lung cancer: a meta-analysis. J Int Med Res 2021;49(9). 3000605211044204.

50. Tane S, Nishio W, Nishioka Y, et al. Evaluation of the Residual Lung Function After Thoracoscopic Segmentectomy Compared With Lobectomy. Ann Thorac Surg 2019;108(5):1543–50.

51. Saito H, Nakagawa T, Ito M, et al. Pulmonary function after lobectomy versus segmentectomy in patients with stage I non-small cell lung cancer. World J Surg 2014;38(8):2025–31.

52. Handa Y, Tsutani Y, Mimae T, et al. Postoperative Pulmonary Function After Complex Segmentectomy. Ann Surg Oncol 2021;28(13):8347–55.

53. Nomori H, Shiraishi A, Yamazaki I, et al. Extent of Segmentectomy That Achieves Greater Lung Preservation Than Lobectomy. Ann Thorac Surg 2021; 112(4):1127–33.

54. Chen L, Gu Z, Lin B, et al. Pulmonary function changes after thoracoscopic lobectomy versus intentional thoracoscopic segmentectomy for early-stage non-small cell lung cancer. Transl Lung Cancer Res 2021;10(11):4141–51.

55. Gu Z, Wang H, Mao T, et al. Pulmonary function changes after different extent of pulmonary resection under video-assisted thoracic surgery. J Thorac Dis 2018;10(4):2331–7.

56. Tao H, Tanaka T, Hayashi T, et al. Influence of stapling the intersegmental planes on lung volume and function after segmentectomy. Interact Cardiovasc Thorac Surg 2016;23(4):548–52.

57. Salazar MC, Canavan ME, Walters SL, et al. The Survival Advantage of Lobectomy over Wedge Resection Lessens as Health-Related Life Expectancy Decreases. JTO Clin Res Rep 2021;2(3):100143.

58. Cao J, Yuan P, Wang Y, et al. Survival Rates After Lobectomy, Segmentectomy, and Wedge Resection for Non-Small Cell Lung Cancer. Ann Thorac Surg 2018;105(5):1483–91.

59. Mimae T, Saji H, Nakamura H, et al. Survival of Octogenarians with Early-Stage Non-small Cell Lung Cancer is Comparable Between Wedge Resection and Lobectomy/Segmentectomy: JACS1303. Ann Surg Oncol 2021;28(12):7219–27.

60. Chan EG, Chan PG, Mazur SN, et al. Outcomes with segmentectomy versus lobectomy in patients with clinical T1cN0M0 non-small cell lung cancer. J Thorac Cardiovasc Surg 2021;161(5):1639–48. e1632.

61. Dolan DP, White A, Mazzola E, et al. Outcomes of superior segmentectomy versus lower lobectomy for superior segment Stage I non-small-cell lung cancer are equivalent: An analysis of 196 patients at a single, high volume institution. J Surg Oncol 2021; 123(2):570–8.

62. Kamel MK, Rahouma M, Lee B, et al. Segmentectomy Is Equivalent to Lobectomy in Hypermetabolic Clinical Stage IA Lung Adenocarcinomas. Ann Thorac Surg 2019;107(1):217–23.

63. Razi SS, Nguyen D, Villamizar N. Lobectomy does not confer survival advantage over segmentectomy for non-small cell lung cancer with unsuspected nodal disease. J Thorac Cardiovasc Surg 2020; 159(6):2469–83.e2464.

64. Bao F, Ye P, Yang Y, et al. Segmentectomy or lobectomy for early stage lung cancer: a meta-analysis. Eur J Cardio Thorac Surg 2014;46(1):1–7.

65. Baig MZ, Razi SS, Muslim Z, et al. Lobectomy demonstrates superior survival than segmentectomy for high-grade non-small cell lung cancer: the national cancer database analysis. Am Surg 2021. 31348211011116.

# Stereotactic Body Radiation Therapy Versus Ablation Versus Surgery for Early-Stage Lung Cancer in High-Risk Patients

Conor M. Maxwell, DO[a],
Calvin Ng, MD (Res) (Lond), FRCSEd, FCSHK, FHKAM (Surg), FCCP, FAPSR[b],
Hiran C. Fernando, MBBS, FRCS[c,*]

KEYWORDS

- SBRT • Thermal ablation • Sublobar resection • Early-stage lung cancer • Segmentectomy
- Wedge resection

KEY POINTS

- Sublobar resection is the preferred approach for patients who can undergo resection—but not tolerate lobectomy.
- When wedge resection is performed, it is important to ensure adequate margins and at a minimum perform lymph node sampling.
- Stereotactic body radiation therapy has shown good results in medically inoperable patients with prospective trials underway to evaluate its role for operable patients.
- Preliminary evidence in thermal ablation and advances in transbronchial approaches such as electromagnetic navigational bronchoscopy and robotic bronchoscopy platforms is showing promise as an effective treatment option and a future direction for medically inoperable patients.

## INTRODUCTION/BACKGROUND

Lung cancer is one of the most common cancers worldwide with more than 2 million new cases a year globally. Unfortunately, it is also the leading cause of cancer-related death, with more deaths than colon, breast, and prostate cancer combined. Most patients with newly diagnosed lung malignancies are already in advanced stages; however, with improved imaging techniques and screening recommendations, an increasing number of patients are being diagnosed earlier. Owing to an aging population, the average age of diagnosis with a new lung mass is approximately 70 years old. Not surprisingly, there is some degree of baseline frailty and therefore, medical inoperability is not uncommon.[1] It is estimated that approximately 20% of patients diagnosed with early-stage non-small cell lung cancer (NSCLC) do not undergo operations related to their comorbid risk factors. Risk factors such as chronic obstructive pulmonary disease (COPD) and heart disease are common comorbid conditions in patients with NSCLC that give them a higher risk status. It should be noted that even in high-risk, medically inoperable patients with early-stage (I to II) lung cancer the median overall survival (OS) if left untreated is 14.2 months with 53% of patients dying from their cancer rather than from other causes.[2]

[a] Department of Surgery, Allegheny General Hospital, 320 East North Avenue, Suite 556, Pittsburgh, PA 15212, USA; [b] Department of Surgery, Prince of Wales Hospital, Shatin, New Territories, Hong Kong; [c] Department of Cardiothoracic Surgery, Allegheny General Hospital, 320 East North Avenue, 14th Floor, South Tower, Pittsburgh, PA 15212, USA
* Corresponding author.
*E-mail address:* Hiran.Fernando@ahn.org

Thorac Surg Clin 33 (2023) 179–187
https://doi.org/10.1016/j.thorsurg.2023.01.003
1547-4127/23/© 2023 Elsevier Inc. All rights reserved.

Current treatment for early-stage lesions focuses on surgical intervention as the mainstay of treatment; however, this poses issues in patients that are unfit to tolerate an operation. In this case, radiation has been the primary treatment for this subset of patients. More recently this has been in the form of stereotactic body radiation therapy (SBRT) also known as stereotactic ablative radiosurgery (SABR). Another approach has been the use of thermal ablation. In this article, we focus on treatment strategies using SBRT, thermal ablation, or surgery as it pertains to high-risk patients with early-stage lung cancer. We will discuss the use of these modalities as a treatment option through an evaluation of current research.

### Patient Evaluation Overview

Patients can be considered in three broad categories, namely (1) standard-risk operable (able to tolerate lobectomy), (2) high-risk operable (lobectomy is considered too high-risk, but the patient can undergo a sublobar resection), and (3) medically inoperable (where a patient is considered too high-risk for any surgical resection). Defining which group patients fall into, can be challenging, but a key component is pulmonary function testing (PFT) and performance status. The American College of Chest Physicians (CHEST) (ACCP) previously addressed this in their guidelines in 2013. They recommended using measurements of Forced Expiratory Volume in 1 second (FEV1) and, carbon monoxide diffusing capacity (DLCO) including predicted postoperative (PPO) lung function estimates to guide the risk assessment for undergoing anatomic resection.[3] Tumor location can also impact this decision. For instance, patients with upper lobe tumors who have upper lobe predominant emphysema may tolerate lung resection well, despite impaired PFT. Overall, the decision of inoperability comes down to a decision between the surgeon and the patient with a thorough explanation of the risks and benefits of each treatment pathway.

### Surgery

Based on the work by Ginsberg and colleagues,[4] lobectomy has been the gold standard management for NSCLC in standard risk operable patients. This randomized study was undertaken in an era where computed tomography (CT) scans were not routine, and all operations were performed by thoracotomy. With the increased adoption of CT scan screening, and identification of smaller lung nodules there has been rekindled interest in the use of segmentectomy for standard-risk patients with small stage I cancers. When

considering high-risk operable patients, sublobar resection, such as segmentectomy or wedge resection has been the standard of care for this subset of patients. Sublobar resection has the benefit of the preservation of postoperative lung function, but still allows resection of cancer with the opportunity for better regional control and cancer staging (compared with nonoperative approaches), as long as lymph node dissection is performed.

Generally, anatomic segmentectomy is considered superior to wedge resection. Margins will tend to be superior, and in addition, dissection of the segmental bronchus, artery, and vein, will lead to better dissection of local N1 lymph nodes. However, there is limited prospective research investigating the difference between methods of sublobar resection. One study by Tsutani and colleagues[5] retrospectively evaluated wedge resection to segmentectomy and found similar OS suggesting that wedge resection is at least equivalent to segmentectomy in patients deemed unfit for surgery. They also found shorter operative times and less blood loss, which is understandably beneficial in a population that is already deemed high risk for an operation. In another study, when comparing sublobar resections, Tsutani and colleagues[6] found better oncologic outcomes after segmentectomy compared to wedge resection, with lower recurrence rates, noting segmentectomy to be a favorable prognostic factor for cumulative incidence of recurrence between the two surgical techniques after propensity matching. Similarly, Handa and colleagues[7] retrospectively analyzed sublobar resections comparing segmentectomy and wedge resection in Stage 1A tumors. Better oncologic outcomes were found in the segmentectomy group with 5-year recurrence-free interval rates of 96.9% versus 87.5%, suggesting that segmentectomy should be performed whenever able in this high-risk population. EL-Sherrif and colleagues[8] reported on 81 stage I NSCLC patients treated with sublobar resection. There were 41 tumors with a surgical margin <1 cm and 40 with a margin>/ = 1 cm. Local recurrence (LR) was significantly ($p = 0.04$) higher at 14.6% in the patients with closer margin than those with wider margins (7.5%). This same study also showed superior ($P = 0.002$) results with segmental resection (LR = 3.8%) compared with wedge resection (LR = 14.5%).

There is a lack of consensus on what constitutes an adequate margin when wedge resection is undertaken. A margin of 1 cm was used in the study discussed above by El-Sherif and colleagues.[8] In a study by Sawabata and colleagues,[9] no relapse was observed on the margin in cases where both negative histology and negative cytology was achieved following run-across cytologic testing of the staple line. This group has further reported a recommendation for obtaining a marginal distance greater than the maximum diameter of the tumor based on further review of positive margins, marginal distance, and tumor size. The margin:tumor ratio was investigated further in a North American series involving 182 patients undergoing segmentectomy.[10] When the margin:tumor ratio was >1, loco-regional recurrence was reduced from 25% to 6.2%. The most recent American College of Chest Physicians (CHEST) guidelines from 2013 suggest resection with a >2 cm margin to minimize LR and for smaller tumors, a margin of at least the diameter of the lesion itself.[3]

## Medically Inoperable

The determination of operability comes down to PFT and multidisciplinary discussion that includes the operating surgeon. An alternative to surgical resection, SBRT is currently indicated for patients that are deemed medically inoperable secondary to comorbid conditions and overall frailty. A newer alternative to SBRT is image-guided thermal ablation (IGTA).

## Stereotactic Body Radiation Therapy

Previously, external beam radiation was the treatment of choice for medically inoperable patients with lung cancer. However, over the past several years, as experience has been gained, and availability of SBRT has increased, this has become the favored approach. This was emphasized in a randomized study comparing SBRT to external beam radiation therapy, where LR rates were doubled in patients receiving external beam radiation.[11] With improved target accuracy and using multiple planes of radiation, much higher radiation doses can be delivered compared with external beam radiation therapy. Traditional external beam radiation treatment plans involving fractions delivered over several weeks may deliver around 60 Gy. SBRT is typically delivered over 1 to 5 fractions. Although dosing is not quite comparable, three doses of 18 Gy delivered by SBRT would deliver a BED of approximately 126 Gy.[12] Many treatment plans allow for a biological effective dose of over 100 Gy and the higher radiation doses provided by SBRT can result in improved local control and survival. For instance, Onishi and colleagues[13] showed that patients who received a dose of <100 Gy (biological equivalent dose) had a 69% survival, whereas those that had a dose > 100 Gy (biological equivalent dose) had an 88% survival at 5 years.

Generally, SBRT has been considered a good option for medically inoperable patients; however, there is increasing interest, particularly among radiation oncologists in using SBRT for high-risk operable as well as standard-risk operable patients. The difference in opinion among specialists was emphasized in a 2018 report of 959 surveys completed by various lung cancer specialists.[14] When asked a series of questions assessing how they felt SBRT compared with surgery given the current state and strength of the evidence, 80% of radiation oncologists responded that SRBT was the same or better than surgery. In contrast, only 28% of nonradiation oncologists surveyed felt that SRBT offered the same or better benefits as compared with surgery. There are several concerns about accepting this view based on currently available literature. These include definitions of LR, lack of tissue diagnosis, and determination of recurrence. It is often wrongly stated that local control is better with SBRT as compared with sublobar resection, and probably equivalent to that of lobectomy. However, the definitions of local control have been different between several surgical and radiation studies. In many radiation studies, local control refers to recurrence only at the irradiated tumor site, essentially a marginal recurrence at the treated tumor site. In addition to marginal recurrence, surgical studies will usually include recurrence in other areas of the lung (eg, in the same lobe but away from the resection site after a wedge resection). In radiation studies, tumor recurrence in another lobe, but in the same lung, will often be considered a distant recurrence, whereas several surgical studies would consider this a locoregional recurrence. In addition, many SBRT studies have included patients who do not have a tissue diagnosis. If a patient never had a malignant tumor, to begin with, and was treated with radiation, estimates of recurrence and cancer-specific survival are meaningless. Finally, PET imaging and biopsy to determine recurrence are often omitted from SBRT studies, so the recurrence may be underestimated. Ideally to make the best evaluation of how SBRT compares with resection, prospective studies with a consistent tissue diagnosis, similar patient populations, and standardized follow-up should be undertaken.

One issue with SBRT is how to determine whether residual tissue remaining after treatment has been completed represents a scar or viable tumor. This was investigated in the MISSLE trial, a phase 2 trial in patients with T1/2N0M0 NSCLC who underwent SBRT followed by resection 10 weeks later. Only 21 (60%) achieved a complete pathologic response when resected.[15] Another interesting propensity-matched analysis from the

National Cancer Database, compared patients who had immediate SBRT (0 to 30 days from diagnosis) to those receiving delayed wedge resection (90 to 120 days from diagnosis). This was an approach suggested by some during the COVID pandemic. Despite a delay in treatment, OS was significantly better after wedge resection.[16] These studies emphasize that in the absence of randomized data, resection should remain the standard for even high-risk operable patients.

Despite largely retrospective data (**Table 1**), a few phase 3 studies to compare SBRT to surgery have been attempted, but none so far have been completed. The randomized study to compare cyberknife to surgical resection in stage I non-small cell lung cancer- NCT00840749 (STARS) and trial of either surgery or stereotactic radiotherapy for early stage (IA) lung cancer- NCT00687986 (ROSEL) trials compared therapy in standard-risk operable patients; however, both trials closed early due to low accrual. A meta-analysis by Chang and colleagues[17] combined and analyzed their data. Although subject to many criticisms, the paper suggested that SBRT was better tolerated and led to 15% better OS compared with surgery for operable clinical stage 1 NSCLC. The total number of patients involved was however very low between the two studies with only 31/1030 accrued in the STARS trial and 27/960 in ROSEL. Therefore, both studies were significantly underpowered. In addition, most of the surgeries were performed via an open approach with a higher surgical mortality rate than typically seen in studies of lobectomy or sublobar resection. Histologic confirmation of NSCLC before treatment was only required in the STARS trial but was not mandatory in the ROSEL trial. For these reasons, the conclusions of the Chang analysis should be interpreted with caution.

Despite the failures to complete prior randomized studies, there are ongoing attempts to study this issue. The veterans affairs lung cancer surgery or stereotactic radiotherapy (VALOR) trial is a prospective, randomized trial in the Veterans population where operable patients are randomized to receive SBRT or surgery in the form of lobectomy or segmentectomy.[18] The primary outcome is OS for up to 10 years with secondary outcomes such as quality of life (QOL), pulmonary function, and local, regional, or distant disease control. The study is estimated to be completed in 2026 and continues to accrue well. Sublobar Resection (SR) Versus Stereotactic Ablative Radiotherapy (SAbR) for Lung Cancer (STABLE-MATES) is another multicenter international trial that compares sublobar resection to SBRT in high-risk operable patients.[19] Currently this study has accrued approximately 75% of its target accrual. It is hoped that these studies will provide better information on which patients are more appropriately treated with SBRT or resection.

Unlike surgery, complications with SBRT typically occur later. Chest wall pain and rib fracture are not uncommon with studies showing fracture rates from 20% to 38%.[20] Radiation-induced pulmonary changes, especially in the form of radiation pneumonitis have also been documented. Pneumonitis rates range from 3% to 11% in most series. A study found 9.4% of patients

**Table 1**
**Surgery versus stereotactic body radiation therapy studies with propensity matching**

| Study | Type | Size (n) Before Matching | Median Survival | 1-Yr Overall Survival (OS) | 3-Yr OS | 5-Yr OS |
|---|---|---|---|---|---|---|
| Dong et al,[38] 2019 | Retrospective, single center | 879 | / | Surgery 98.5% SBRT 98.5% | Surgery 89.4% SBRT 83.9% | / |
| Detillon et al,[39] 2019 | Retrospective, registry center | 792 | Surgery 77 mths SBRT 38 mths | Surgery 91% SBRT 87% | Surgery 68% SBRT 46% | Surgery 58% SBRT 29% |
| Cornwell et al,[40] 2018 | Retrospective, single center | 183 | Surgery >8 yrs SBRT 3.1 yrs | Surgery 94.6 SBRT 89.2 | Surgery 85.7, SBRT 52.9% | / |
| Lin et al,[41] 2019 | Retrospective, single center | 316 | / | / | Surgery 78.5% SBRT 79.5% | / |
| Hamaji et al,[42] 2015 | Retrospective, single center | 517 | / | / | / | Surgery 68.5% SBRT 37.3% |

developed grade 2 to 4 pneumonitis with the majority (7%) being self-limited grade 2 toxicity.[21] Toxicities such as fistula, bronchial stricture, pneumothorax, and hemoptysis are less common. This highlights the importance of patient-tailored regimens based on factors such as presence of osteoporosis, tumor location in close proximity to the chest wall or hilum, and tumor dimensions to limit healthy tissue radiation as much as possible.

## Thermal Ablation

IGTA is an option that has gained popularity among some thoracic and interventional radiology groups. These procedures are largely performed by CT guidance. IGTA is part of the current NCCN guidelines as a treatment option for medically inoperable patients with stage 1 NSCLC. Different modalities of treatment include radiofrequency ablation (RFA), microwave ablation (MVA), and cryoablation (CRA). The benefits of IGTA in high-risk populations are its ability to be performed under conscious sedation.

## Radiofrequency Ablation

RFA for percutaneous tumor ablation was first introduced in the early 1990s and has since been researched as a treatment of cancers such as those of the liver, breast, prostate, and kidney. RFA functions by inducing coagulative necrosis by heating the surrounding tissue to a temperature >60°C.[22] One of the benefits of RFA is that the lungs provide an optimal environment for ablation as parenchyma provides good demarcation between tumor and normal aerated lung to ensure precise location for needle and probe deployment. An issue that can impact the effectiveness of ablation is the "heat sink" effect whereby blood vessels and large airways in proximity to the target site can decrease the effect, by conducting heat away from the tumor. Studies have shown higher rates of LR with treated tumors adjacent to vessels greater than 3 mm.[23]

Dupuy and colleagues[24] performed RFA percutaneously on 54 patients with 1A NSCLC that were deemed high risk for resection after evaluation by a board-certified thoracic surgeon. Patients were followed at 3, 6, 9, 12, 18, and 24 months postprocedure. Of the 54 enrolled patients, 37 completed follow-up, and 15 patients died during the 2-year follow-up period. OS at 1 and 2 years was 86.5% and 71.2%, respectively. There was a 71.2% LR free rate. Significant adverse events described as grade 3 to 5 were encountered at a rate of 11.5% which is comparable to other studies. There were no grade 4 or 5 adverse events. Most of the adverse events were

pneumothoraces that required chest tube placement. In one study comparing SBRT to RFA, RFA showed better OS and cancer-specific survival when used for Stage1A NSCLC.[25]

Although there have been concerns regarding the risks of pneumothorax in high-risk patients, there does not seem to be a significant impact on pulmonary function. The Radiofrequency Ablation of Pulmonary Tumors Response Evaluation (RAPTURE) trial studying the safety and efficacy of RFA found no significant worsening of pulmonary function following ablation.[26] In addition in the prospective Alliance study described above, there was no significant difference in pulmonary function at follow-up.

## Microwave ablation (MWA)

MVA creates a zone of tissue ablation by emitting electromagnetic waves that cause oscillation of surrounding water molecules, friction, and thus heat. Unlike RFA, this technique is less affected by the "heat sink" effect. It has been shown to create more uniform ablation patterns in a shorter period. Studies in patients with hepatocellular carcinoma found MVA to require fewer needle punctures, shorter treatment times, and even lower hospitalization costs when compared with RFA.[27] MWA is rapidly becoming a favored ablative approach for lung cancer. However, minimal prospective comparisons to RFA for lung cancer have not been undertaken. Ni and colleagues[28] studied long-term follow-up over approximately 4 years in 105 patients that underwent MVA for treatment of NSCLC. OS was 99% at 1 year, 75.6% at 3 years, and 54.1% at 5 years, whereas cancer-specific survival rates were 99%, 78.9%, and 60.9%, respectively. Treated 1 A lesions had significantly better DFS and OS than 1B tumors.

## Cryoablation

CRA uses freeze/thaw cycles to promote intracellular ice crystal formation, organelle and cell wall disruption, microvascular thrombosis, and thus cell death.[29] The benefit of CRA that makes it suitable for treating lung tumors is that due to the freeze/thaw process, structures made up of a collagenous matrix such as blood vessels, and bronchi remain intact, making it ideal for central tumors especially those near the hilum. CRA has acceptable rates of complications that are similar to other IGTA modalities. Pneumothorax, pleural effusion, and hemoptysis remain the most common post-procedural complications.[30] Moore and colleagues[31] found 5-year OS of 67.8% and Cancer specific survival (CSS) of 56.6% following percutaneous CRA on 45 patients with early-

**Table 2**
**Image-guided thermal ablation studies in lung cancer**

| IGTA Technique | Study | Study Type | Study Size (n) | 1-y Overall Survival | 3-y Overall Survival | 5-y Overall Survival |
|---|---|---|---|---|---|---|
| Cryo | Moore et al,[31] 2015 | Retrospective | 45 | / | / | 68% |
|  | Kawamura et al,[43] 2006 | Retrospective | 20 | 89% | / | / |
|  | Yamauchi et al,[44] 2012 | Retrospective | 22 | / | 88% | / |
| MWA | Ni et al,[28] 2022 | Retrospective | 105 | 99% | 76% | 54% |
|  | Healey et al,[45] 2017 | Retrospective | 108 | 89%[a] | 75%[a] | 57%[a] |
|  | Yang et al,[46] 2014 | Retrospective | 47 | 89% | 43% | 16% |
| RFA | Dupuy et al,[24] 2015 | Prospective, multicenter | 54 | 86% | / | / |
|  | Palussière et al,[47] 2018 | Prospective Phase 2 multicenter | 32 | 92% | 58% | / |
|  | Simon et al,[48] 2007 | Retrospective | 153 | 78% | 36% | 27% |
|  | Lencioni et al,[26] 2008 | Prospective, multicenter | 106 | 70% | / | / |

[a] Actuarial overall survival.

stage lung cancer that were deemed medically inoperable. Major complications occurred in 6.4% of patients. When comparing CRA to MWA, significantly higher post-procedural pain scores were found in patients with MWA when compared with patients undergoing CRA. OS, local and distant recurrence were similar between the two groups.[32] An advantage of cryotherapy is that an ice ball will occur as the ablation is being delivered. The ice-ball development can be followed in real-time with CT imaging, which is helpful in monitoring the progress of treatment. A disadvantage with the CRA and some of the available MWA systems is that multiple applicators are required for the successful ablation of tumors. It can be challenging to place multiple probes simultaneously into pulmonary tumors in an appropriate orientation because of displacement by the ribs around the tumor. Reported experience with CRA for lung cancer is still relatively limited in comparison to the other thermal ablation modalities (**Table 2**).

## Future Directions

Since the first landmark trials in thoracic surgery, such as those by Ginsberg and colleagues[4] there have been vast advances in screening and management of thoracic malignancies. This landscape continues to change as different treatment modalities are designed. One such treatment option that has shown promising results in early studies is the utilization of a transbronchial approach to IGTA. Percutaneous approaches have been associated with complications such as bronchopleural fistula,

pneumothorax, and hemothorax in certain studies. A transbronchial approach offers the benefit of potentially decreasing these risks as well as accessing tumors not amendable to percutaneous methods such as those with more central orientation, or tumors blocked by the scapula or near the apex for example, as well as numerous pulmonary lesions to be treated in the same session.[33] Ishiwata and colleagues[34] performed RFA by using endobronchial ultrasound in five patients (5 total lesions). Endobronchial Ultrasound (EBUS) was used to localize the lesion and an RFA probe was placed

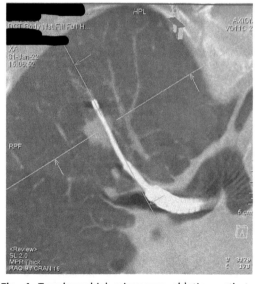

**Fig. 1.** Transbronchial microwave ablation catheter deployed into right upper lobe 1.5-cm NSCLC.

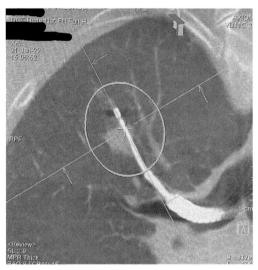

**Fig. 2.** Predicted ablation zone (*green circle*) of 3.5 cm × 4.2 cm with 100 W 10 min of ablation.

within the nodule through the working port of the bronchoscope. Following ablation, bronchoscopy and CT scan were performed to evaluate treatment efficacy and for possible complications. The procedure was well tolerated and on pathologic examination determined a mean ablation zone of 1.8 cm. Chan and colleagues[35] used electromagnetic navigational bronchoscopy to accurately map the lung and successfully microwave ablate tumors in 30 patients. Only 2 patients developed a pneumothorax and post-procedural pain was only experienced in 13% of patients. Lau and colleagues[36] performed bronchoscopic MWA on 30 subjects, the majority

of which were peripheral tumors. They found a technical success of 100% with no 30-day progression. They had no deaths and complications were low including zero pneumothoraxes. All treated nodules were <3 cm and follow-up occurred over 30 days. The results of this study have not yet been published. A group from China is in the recruiting phase to prospectively study MVA versus RFA in medically inoperable patients.[37] Navigational bronchoscopy will be used to aid in bronchoscopic guidance. The primary outcome of the study is local control; however, OS, disease-free survival, and progression-free survival will also be reported. With newer robotic bronchoscopy platforms becoming prominent, we anticipate that this will continue to play a larger role in IGTA, allowing for more precise localization and treatment of lesions (**Figs. 1–3**).

## SUMMARY

In standard-risk operable patients, lobectomy should continue to be the primary treatment offered. However, based on the results of recent randomized trials, segmentectomy may be reasonable for peripheral tumors 2 cm or less. Otherwise, sublobar resection (preferentially segmentectomy, should be reserved for high-risk operable patients). SBRT is a good choice for medically inoperable patients. SBRT may have a role in some high-risk operable patients, and the current ongoing randomized trials will help define this further. IGTA remains a good option for medically inoperable patients, but supportive data comparing this to SBRT is lacking. Bronchoscopic ablation is a new approach that has the potential to replace percutaneous IGTA in the future.

## CLINICS CARE POINTS

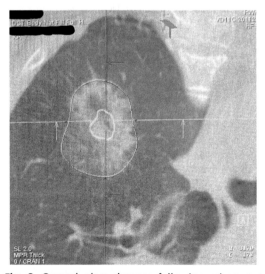

**Fig. 3.** Ground glass changes following microwave ablation covering the tumor that is no longer clearly visible (*yellow outline* from prior CT image overlay), with good margins.

- For patients able to tolerate surgical resection, lobectomy with lymph node sampling remains the gold standard management
- Segmentectomy is a viable option in patients with small primary tumors with similar morbidity/mortality and survival to lobectomy
- Sublobar resection is the preferred approach for patients who can undergo resection—but not lobectomy
- Care should be taken to ensure adequate margins during wedge resection with lymph node sampling if able
- Stereotactic body radiation therapy has shown promise as an alternative to surgery in high-risk patients with prospective trials underway

- Preliminary evidence in image-guided thermal ablation and advances in transbronchial approaches such as electromagnetic navigational bronchoscopy and robotic bronchoscopy platforms are showing promise as an effective treatment option and as a future direction for medically inoperable patients

## REFERENCES

1. American Cancer Society. Cancer Statistics Center. Available at: http://cancerstatisticscenter.cancer.org. Accessed June 6, 2022.
2. McGarry RC, Song G, des Rosiers P, et al. Observation-only management of early stage, medically inoperable lung cancer: poor outcome. Chest 2002;121(4):1155–8.
3. Detterbeck FC, Lewis SZ, Diekemper R, et al. Executive Summary: Diagnosis and management of lung cancer, 3rd ed: American College of Chest Physicians evidence-based clinical practice guidelines. Chest 2013;143(5 Suppl):7S–37S.
4. Ginsberg RJ, Rubinstein LV. Randomized trial of lobectomy versus limited resection for T1 N0 non-small cell lung cancer. Lung Cancer Study Group. Ann Thorac Surg 1995;60(3):615–23.
5. Tsutani Y, Kagimoto A, Handa Y, et al. Wedge resection versus segmentectomy in patients with stage I non-small-cell lung cancer unfit for lobectomy. Japanese journal of clinical oncology. Available at: https://pubmed.ncbi.nlm.nih.gov/31602468/. Published December 27, 2019. Accessed July 19, 2022.
6. Tsutani Y, Handa Y, Shimada Y, et al. Comparison of cancer control between segmentectomy and wedge resection in patients with clinical stage IA non–small cell lung cancer. The Journal of Thoracic and Cardiovascular Surgery. Available at: https://www.sciencedirect.com/science/article/abs/pii/S0022522320328336. Published October 22, 2020. Accessed July 19, 2022.
7. Handa Y, Tsutani Y, Mimae T, et al. A Multicenter Study of Complex Segmentectomy Versus Wedge Resection in Clinical Stage 0-IA Non-Small Cell Lung Cancer. Clin Lung Cancer 2022;23(5):393–401.
8. El-Sherif A, Fernando HC, Santos R, et al. Margin and local recurrence after sublobar resection of non-small cell lung cancer. Ann Surg Oncol 2007;14(8):2400–5.
9. Sawabata N, Matsumura A, Ohota M, et al. Cytologically malignant margins of wedge resected stage I non-small cell lung cancer. Ann Thorac Surg 2002;74(6):1953–7.
10. Schuchert MJ, Pettiford BL, Keeley S, et al. Anatomic segmentectomy in the treatment of stage I non-small cell lung cancer. Ann Thorac Surg 2007;84(3):926–33.
11. Ball D, Mai GT, Vinod S, et al. Stereotactic ablative radiotherapy versus standard radiotherapy in stage 1 non-small-cell lung cancer (TROG 09.02 CHISEL): a phase 3, open-label, randomised controlled trial. Lancet Oncol 2019;20(4):494–503.
12. Macià I Garau M. Radiobiology of stereotactic body radiation therapy (SBRT). Rep Pract Oncol Radiother 2017;22(2):86–95.
13. Onishi H, Araki T, Shirato H, et al. Stereotactic hypofractionated high-dose irradiation for stage I non-small cell lung carcinoma: clinical outcomes in 245 subjects in a Japanese multiinstitutional study. Cancer 2004;101(7):1623–31.
14. Lammers A, Mitin T, Moghanaki D, et al. Lung cancer specialists' opinions on treatment for stage I non-small cell lung cancer: A multidisciplinary survey. Adv Radiat Oncol 2018;3(2):125–9.
15. Palma DA, Nguyen TK, Louie AV, et al. Measuring the Integration of Stereotactic Ablative Radiotherapy Plus Surgery for Early-Stage Non-Small Cell Lung Cancer: A Phase 2 Clinical Trial. JAMA Oncol 2019;5(5):681–8.
16. Mayne NR, Lin BK, Darling AJ, et al. Stereotactic Body Radiotherapy Versus Delayed Surgery for Early-stage Non-small-cell Lung Cancer. Ann Surg 2020;272(6):925–9.
17. Chang JY, Senan S, Paul MA, et al. Stereotactic ablative radiotherapy versus lobectomy for operable stage I non-small-cell lung cancer: a pooled analysis of two randomised trials. Lancet Oncol 2015;16(6):630–7 [published correction appears in Lancet Oncol. 2015 Sep;16(9):e427].
18. Cameron R, Gage D. Veterans Affairs Lung Cancer Surgery Or Stereotactic Radiotherapy Trial (VALOR). ClinicalTrials.gov identifier: NCT02984761. Available at: https://clinicaltrials.gov/ct2/show/NCT02984761. Updated March 21, 2022. Accessed July 19, 2022.
19. Teke ME, Sarvestani AL, Hernandez JM, et al. A Randomized, Phase III Study of Sublobar Resection (SR) Versus Stereotactic Ablative Radiotherapy (SAbR) in High-Risk Patients with Stage I Non-Small Cell Lung Cancer (NSCLC). Ann Surg Oncol 2022;29(8):4686–7.
20. Thibault I, Chiang A, Erler D, et al. Predictors of Chest Wall Toxicity after Lung Stereotactic Ablative Radiotherapy. Clin Oncol 2016;28(1):28–35.
21. Barriger RB, Forquer JA, Brabham JG, et al. A dose-volume analysis of radiation pneumonitis in non-small cell lung cancer patients treated with stereotactic body radiation therapy. Int J Radiat Oncol Biol Phys 2012;82(1):457–62.
22. Ridge CA, Solomon SB, Thornton RH. Thermal ablation of stage I non-small cell lung carcinoma. Semin Intervent Radiol 2014;31(2):118–24.

23. Gillams AR, Lees WR. Radiofrequency ablation of lung metastases: factors influencing success. Eur Radiol 2008;18(4):672–7.

24. Dupuy DE, Fernando HC, Hillman S, et al. Radiofrequency ablation of stage IA non-small cell lung cancer in medically inoperable patients: Results from the American College of Surgeons Oncology Group Z4033 (Alliance) trial. Cancer 2015;121(19):3491–8.

25. Li M, Xu X, Qin Y, et al. Radiofrequency ablation *vs.* stereotactic body radiotherapy for stage IA non-small cell lung cancer in nonsurgical patients. J Cancer 2021;12(10):3057–66.

26. Lencioni R, Crocetti L, Cioni R, et al. Response to radiofrequency ablation of pulmonary tumours: a prospective, intention-to-treat, multicentre clinical trial (the RAPTURE study). Lancet Oncol 2008;9(7):621–8.

27. Yu J, Yu XL, Han ZY, et al. Percutaneous cooled-probe microwave versus radiofrequency ablation in early-stage hepatocellular carcinoma: a phase III randomised controlled trial. Gut 2017;66(6):1172–3.

28. Ni Y, Huang G, Yang X, et al. Microwave ablation treatment for medically inoperable stage I non-small cell lung cancers: long-term results. Eur Radiol 2022;32(8):5616–22.

29. Whittaker DK. Mechanisms of tissue destruction following cryosurgery. Ann R Coll Surg Engl 1984;66(5):313–8.

30. Inoue M, Nakatsuka S, Yashiro H, et al. Percutaneous cryoablation of lung tumors: feasibility and safety. J Vasc Interv Radiol 2012;23(3):295–305.

31. Moore W, Talati R, Bhattacharji P, et al. Five-year survival after cryoablation of stage I non-small cell lung cancer in medically inoperable patients. J Vasc Interv Radiol 2015;26(3):312–9.

32. Li HW, Long YJ, Yan GW, et al. Microwave ablation vs. cryoablation for treatment of primary and metastatic pulmonary malignant tumors. Mol Clin Oncol 2022;16(3):62.

33. Chan JWY, Lau RWH, Chang A, et al. Transbronchial Microwave Ablation – Important Role in the Battle of Lung Preservation for Multifocal Lung Primaries or Metastases. *Ann Oncol.* April 2022;33(Suppl 2):S76–7.

34. Ishiwata T, Motooka Y, Ujiie H, et al. Endobronchial ultrasound-guided bipolar radiofrequency ablation for lung cancer: A first-in human clinical trial [published online ahead of print, 2022 Mar 26]. J Thorac Cardiovasc Surg 2022;S0022-5223(22):00344-350.

35. Chan JWY, Lau RWH, Ngai JCL, et al. Transbronchial microwave ablation of lung nodules with electromagnetic navigation bronchoscopy guidance-a novel technique and initial experience with 30 cases. Transl Lung Cancer Res 2021;10(4):1608–22.

36. Lau K, Lau R, Baranowski R, et al. Late breaking abstract - bronchoscopic microwave ablation of peripheral lung tumors. European Respiratory Society. Available at: https://erj.ersjournals.com/content/58/suppl_65/OA230. Published September 5, 2021.

37. Sun J. Transbronchial Ablation for Peripheral Lung Tumor. ClinicalTrials.gov identifier: NCT02972177. Available at: https://clinicaltrials.gov/ct2/show/NCT02972177. Updated February 18,2020. Accessed July 2, 2022.

38. Dong B, Wang J, Xu Y, et al. Comparison of the Efficacy of Stereotactic Body Radiotherapy versus Surgical Treatment for Early-Stage Non-Small Cell Lung Cancer after Propensity Score Matching. Transl Oncol 2019;12(8):1032–7.

39. Detillon DDEMA, Aarts MJ, De Jaeger K, et al. Video-assisted thoracic lobectomy *versus* stereotactic body radiotherapy for stage I nonsmall cell lung cancer in elderly patients: a propensity matched comparative analysis. Eur Respir J 2019;53(6):1801561.

40. Cornwell LD, Echeverria AE, Samuelian J, et al. Video-assisted thoracoscopic lobectomy is associated with greater recurrence-free survival than stereotactic body radiotherapy for clinical stage I lung cancer. J Thorac Cardiovasc Surg 2018;155(1):395–402.

41. Lin Q, Sun X, Zhou N, et al. Outcomes of stereotactic body radiotherapy versus lobectomy for stage I non-small cell lung cancer: a propensity score matching analysis. BMC Pulm Med 2019;19(1):98.

42. Hamaji M, Chen F, Matsuo Y, et al. Video-assisted thoracoscopic lobectomy versus stereotactic radiotherapy for stage I lung cancer. Ann Thorac Surg 2015;99(4):1122–9.

43. Kawamura M, Izumi Y, Tsukada N, et al. Percutaneous cryoablation of small pulmonary malignant tumors under computed tomographic guidance with local anesthesia for nonsurgical candidates. J Thorac Cardiovasc Surg 2006;131(5):1007–13.

44. Yamauchi Y, Izumi Y, Hashimoto K, et al. Percutaneous cryoablation for the treatment of medically inoperable stage I non-small cell lung cancer. PLoS One 2012;7(3):e33223.

45. Healey TT, March BT, Baird G, et al. Microwave Ablation for Lung Neoplasms: A Retrospective Analysis of Long-Term Results. J Vasc Interv Radiol 2017;28(2):206–11.

46. Yang X, Ye X, Zheng A, et al. Percutaneous microwave ablation of stage I medically inoperable non-small cell lung cancer: clinical evaluation of 47 cases. J Surg Oncol 2014;110(6):758–63.

47. Palussière J, Chomy F, Savina M, et al. Radiofrequency ablation of stage IA non-small cell lung cancer in patients ineligible for surgery: results of a prospective multicenter phase II trial. J Cardiothorac Surg 2018;13(1):91.

48. Simon CJ, Dupuy DE, DiPetrillo TA, et al. Pulmonary radiofrequency ablation: long-term safety and efficacy in 153 patients. Radiology 2007;243(1):268–75.

# Current Management of Stage IIIA (N2) Non-Small-Cell Lung Cancer

## Role of Perioperative Immunotherapy, and Tyrosine Kinase Inhibitors

Darren S. Bryan, MD, Jessica S. Donington, MD*

### KEYWORDS

- Non-small-cell lung cancer • Surgery • Stage III • Induction therapy • Immunotherapy
- Multimodality therapy

### KEY POINTS

- Stage III non-small-cell lung cancer encompasses a heterogenous population of patients and the role of surgery is dictated by the bulk and extent of the nodal involvement.
- Recent trials show promising survival with the integration of targeted and immunotherapies into perioperative care for stage IIIA non-small-cell lung cancer.
- Immunotherapies and targeted therapies have received regulatory approval for use in resectable non-small-cell lung cancer-based on trials with pathologic and recurrence-based primary endpoints and before evidence for an overall survival benefit.
- Early surgical safety data related to neoadjuvant chemoimmunotherapy may broaden the population of stage IIIA patients considered for surgical resection.
- Recent neoadjuvant trials show significant regional variability related to attrition, pneumonectomy use, and rates of R0 resection that suggest variability in surgical decision-making in stage IIIA disease.

## INTRODUCTION

Treatment paradigms in non-small-cell lung cancer (NSCLC) have evolved substantially over the past 5 years. Although lung cancer remains responsible for the majority of cancer deaths worldwide, immune checkpoint inhibitors (ICIs), and targeted therapies have opened new treatment pathways with encouraging early results.[1,2] Surgical resection alone remains a curative intent treatment strategy for earliest-stage patients with survival in >70%; however, locally advanced disease has historically seen far lower survival and multimodal treatment.[3]

Stage III is a pathologically diverse entity subdivided into IIIA, IIIB, and IIIC classifications in the 8th edition of the American Joint Committee on Cancer's (AJCC) TNM staging system.[4] Patients with IIIB and IIIC disease, characterized by N3 nodal involvement or N2 nodal involvement with large (T3 or T4) primary tumors, are not generally approached surgically. Stage IIIA NSCLC is a particularly heterogenous group with regard to disease extent and treatment. Stage IIIA encompasses patients with large tumors and no mediastinal nodal involvement (T3N1, T4N0-1), and smaller tumors with N2 nodal involvement (T1-2N2). Curative-intent treatment therefore

Dr J.S. Donington serves as a speaker and advisor for AstraZeneca, BMS, Roche/Genentech and Merck.
Section of Thoracic Surgery, Department of Surgery, University of Chicago Medicine, Room S-546/MC 5047, 5841 South Maryland Avenue, Chicago, IL 60637, USA
* Corresponding author.
*E-mail address:* jdonington@uchicago.edu

Thorac Surg Clin 33 (2023) 189–196
https://doi.org/10.1016/j.thorsurg.2023.01.006
1547-4127/23/© 2023 Elsevier Inc. All rights reserved.

requires a nuanced approach, combining local and systemic therapies. Here, we review the rapidly evolving data for the use of ICIs and targeted therapy in the treatment of stage IIIA NSCLC, as well as long-standing surgical controversies in the treatment of IIIA disease.

## RECENT ADVANCES IN LOCALLY RESECTABLE NON-SMALL-CELL LUNG CANCER
### Adjuvant Immunotherapy

In patients with advanced NSCLC, ICI and targeted therapy have been shown to improve progression-free survival (PFS) and overall survival (OS) in select populations.[5–10] In 2017, the landmark PACIFIC trial showed improved PFS in patients with unresectable stage III NSCLC treated with adjuvant consolidation durvalumab as compared to placebo (hazard ratio [HR] 0.52; 95% confidence interval [CI], 0.42 to 0.65).[11] In 2018, a significcnat OS benefit was also reported.[12] Starting in 2020, phase III studies began reporting improved survival outcomes for ICI and epidermal growth factor receptor (EGFR)-targeted therapy in the adjuvant setting in patients with resectable stage III diseas

IMpower010 was the first randomized, Phase III multicenter trial to report benefits of ICIs in the adjuvant setting. A total of 1005 patients with completely resected stage IB-IIIA NSCLC who had completed at least one cycle of adjuvant platinum-based chemotherapy were randomized to atezolizumab, an anti-programmed death-ligand 1 (PD-L1) monoclonal antibody, versus best supportive care. The atezolizumab arm did not cross statistical significance in the intention to treat the population of patients with stage IB to IIIA disease (HR 0.81; 95% CI, 0.67 to 0.99), but a statistically significant disease-free survival (DFS) benefit (HR 0.66; 95% CI, 0.5 to 0.88) was found in the stage II to IIIA population expressing PD-L1 on ≥ 1% of cells, leading to regulatory approval in the United States for patients with ≥1% PD-L1 expression. Subgroup analysis showed that much of this benefit was driven by patients with high PD-L1 expression (≥50% of cells, HR 0.42; 95% CI, 0.27 to 0.68), and in Europe and Canada regulatory approval was only granted for tumors with ≥50% PD-L1 expression.[13] Early OS data for Impower010 presented at the World Conference for Lung Cancer (WCLC) in the summer of 2022 showed significant benefit with the addition of atezolizumab for high expressing tumors at 3 years (HR 0.42; 95% CI, 0.23 to 0.78) but not for the broader PD-L1 population (HR 0.67; 95% CI, 0.45 to 0.98) decreasing some enthusiasm for adding adjuvant atezolizumab for tumors with PD-L1 expression in 1% to 49% of cells.[14]

Results from KEYNOTE-091 (PEARLS) trial added some confusion to the adjuvant ICI picture. It was also a multicenter phase III trial, randomizing patients with stage IB-IIIA NSCLC to adjuvant pembrolizumab, an anti- PD-1, or placebo, but adjuvant chemotherapy was optional. Unlike IMpower010, the treatment arm showed significant improvement in DFS in the intention to treat population (HR 0.76; 95% CI, 0.63 to 0.91); however, DFS was not significantly imporved in PD-L1 high expressing tumors.[15] OS for this trial has yet to be reported. It is unclear if the differential survival outcomes between PEARLS and Impower010 are due to the efficacy of PD-L1 versus PD-1 antibodies, a result of optional chemotherapy, or simply a reflection of an unreliability of the PD-L1 biomarker.

### Adjuvant Targeted Therapies

Various targeted molecular therapies have been investigated for the treatment of metastatic NSCLC, including those targeting mutations to BRAF serine/threonine-protein kinase (BRAF), anaplastic lymphoma kinase (ALK), MET proto-oncogene, receptor tyrosine kinase (MET), rearranged during transfection or ret proto-oncogene (RET), Kirsten rat sarcoma viral oncogene homolog (KRAS), ROS protooncogene 1, receptor tyrosine kinase (ROS1), neurotrophic tropomyosin recpetor kinase gene fusion (NTREK), and EGFR. Oncogenic driver mutations to the tyrosine kinase domain of the EGFR gene are commonly encountered, occurring in approximately 10% to 15% of North American and Western Europe patients, and 30% to 50% of East Asian populations.[16] Extensive research has focused on the most common mutations within EGFR, occurring in exons 18-21.[17,18] The third-generation EGFR tyrosine kinase inhibitor (TKI), osimertinib, is now standard-of-care first-line therapy for advanced-stage EGFR-mutant NSCLC, based on results from the FLAURA trial with longer PFS and OS when compared to earlier generation TKIs.[10] Expanding on those results, the ADAURA trial randomized patients with completely resected stage IB-IIIA EGFR-mutated NSCLC to 3 years of adjuvant osimertinib or placebo. Results were unblinded early when Data Safety Monitoring Board noted a significant 2-year DFS benefit for patients with stage II-IIIA disease, 90% versus 44% for treatment versus placebo arms, representing a magnitude of benefit rarely seen in oncologic trials (HR, 0.17, 95% CI, 0.11 to 0.26).[19] Updated ADAURA data were reported at WCLC in 2022. Although there seems to be some increase in disease recurrence in the Osimertinib arm following the completion of therapy, the impressive DFS benefit persists through 4 years in the resected II to IIIA population (HR 0.23; 95% CI, 0.18 to 0.30).[20] These results have changed the treatment paradigm for early-stage EGFR-mutated patients.

### Neoadjuvant Chemo-Immunotherapy

ICIs have also been applied in the neoadjuvant setting for locally advanced NSCLC, as a result of practice-changing trials reported in the past 2 years. CheckMate 816 investigated the use of neoadjuvant nivolumab, an anti-PD-1 monoclonal antibody, plus platinum-based chemotherapy versus neoadjuvant chemotherapy alone in patients with resectable stage IB-IIIA NSCLC. The trial reported significantly longer event-free survival (EFS), 31.6 months versus 20.8 months (HR 0.63; 97.38% CI, 0.43 to 0.91), as well as an impressive improvement in the rate of pathologic complete response (pCR) in the treatment arm (24% vs 2%, OR 13.94).[21] Patients with stage IIIA disease (HR 0.54), and those with PD-L1 expressed on ≥1% of tumor cells (HR 0.41) showed the greatest improvements in EFS. Regulatory approval for nivolumab in combination with platinum-doublet chemotherapy in the neoadjuvant setting was granted based on these results.

The NADIM II trial was also reported in 2022 and further supporting the benefit of neoadjuvant chemo-immunotherapy. This smaller trial randomized 90 patients with resectable stage IIIA and IIIB NSCLC to neoadjuvant nivolumab plus platinum-based chemotherapy versus chemotherapy alone. Those who went on to R0 resections received adjuvant nivolumab for six months. pCR rates were significantly increased with the addition of ICI (36.2% vs 6.8%, response rate [RR] 5.25; 95% CI, 1.32 to 20.87).[22] At a planned 24-month data cutoff reported at the 2022 WCLC, OS was significantly longer in the nivolumab group (85.3% vs 64.8%, HR 0.37; 95% CI,0.14 to 0.93), with particular benefit in patients with ≥1% PD-L1 expression (HR 0.26; 95% CI, 0.08 to 0.77).[23]

### CONTROVERSIES IN STAGE III DISEASE

The addition of targeted therapies and ICI represents a significant advancement for patients with early and locally advanced NSCLC but has not simplified treatment decisions. Tumor biomarkers help to direct treatment, but many long-standing controversies related to surgery in this population persist. Successful treatment of stage III lung cancer requires a combination of both systemic and local therapies. Although systemic treatment is needed to decrease the risk of distant disease, extirpation of the primary tumor is essential for cure. The role of surgery in stage IIIB and IIIC is limited, although the 8th edition of AJCC NSCLC staging moved T4N2 tumors to stage IIIB and a subset of these tumors are potentially resectable. Surgery is an important treatment option for a significant subset of patients with IIIA disease.

### Are Recurrence-Based Survival Endpoints Sufficient to Change Practice?

An initial controversy to consider regarding the recent important adjuvant and neoadjuvant trials is whether their results should change practice without evidence for improvements in OS. The gold standard for outcome measurement in oncology trials in curative populations is OS, but it is slow to mature and difficult to measure in curative cohorts. Surrogate endpoints that are recurrence-based, such as DFS and EFS, have been the primary endpoints in the recently reported adjuvant and neoadjuvant ICI and targeted therapy trials with the goal of early identification of important differences in treatment that may predate a reportable OS advantage. Only the Impower010 trial has reported OS data and the advantage was in a select population [PD-L1 >50%, stage II-IIIA(HR 0.42; 95%CI,0.23 to 0.78)].[14] The central question with recurrence-based endpoints is whether the additional therapies are truly curing patients or just delaying recurrence. This may be related to the agents being investigated and the magnitude of the benefit in recurrence. It may be hard to establish OS benefit to adjuvant Osimertinib from the ADURA trial, as no trial in stage IV disease has ever shown an OS benefit for use of an EGFR-TKI, but the dramatic reduction in disease recurrence appears to be enough to change practice, regardless of an OS benefit. Conversely, the landmark PACIFIC trial reported significant PFS improvements with adjuvant durvalumab in 2017 and received FDA approval based on that finding, 5 years before the 2022 report of significant OS (47.5 vs 29.1 months).[11,12,24] The PFS benefit was stable over time and translated to an OS benefit. Two different classes of agnets with differing modes of tumor control.

Pathologic endpoints, such as pCR rate and major pathologic response rate (MPR) are frequent primary endpoints in recently reported and ongoing neoadjuvant chemo-immunotherapy trials. A major advantage of these endpoints is speed—they are available at the time of resection and are considered to be indicative of the magnitude of response, but a clear correlation with OS has yet to be firmly established in NSCLC.

### Defining resectability

Treatment decisions on operability for IIIA patients depend primarily upon the extent of nodal involvement, extent of the indicated operation, patient performance status, and provider expertise. N2 involvement is the defining feature for most stage IIIA patients. The current staging system does not take into account the extent of nodal involvement, it does not differentiate between small-volume disease and that which is extensive, bulky, or infiltrative. There have been attempts to further classify nodal involvement as that which is incidental or occult (unknown at the time of resection and often not detected on preoperative imaging or pathologic assessment), clinically identified preoperatively and considered to be resectable (poorly defined, however frequently single station nodal disease, not invasive into surrounding structures), and nodal involvement rendering patients unresectable (bulky, multistation, or infiltrative).[25]

Although many consider single-station N2 disease to be potentially resectable, opinions are far more mixed on the role of surgery for multistation or bulky N2 involvement, with some biases rooted in specialty. A 2012 study of medical oncologists showed that 92% believed surgery to be an important component of multimodal care for occult and single station N2-positive IIIA disease, whereas fewer than 50% believed surgery to be advisable if N2 disease were considered to be "bulky or multistation".26

### Do the CheckMate-816 results change definition of resectable disease?

One must question if the results from CheckMate 816 will change the definition for resectable IIIA NSCLC. More than 60% of patients enrolled on CheckMate 816 had stage IIIA disease and the trial noted trends toward shorter average operative time, less blood loss, more minimally invasive procedures, and fewer pneumonectomies, suggesting potentially easier operations due to extent of disease response with the addition of nivolumab to induction chemotherapy. Furthermore, pathologic downstaging and pCR were significantly more common. These factors, along with improved EFS, have led many to consider the potential benefit of a surgical approach to stage IIIA disease. Time will tell if the impressive pCR rates operative results from the induction chemo-immunotherapy trials will expand the pool of providers willing to consider a surgical approach to non-bulky multi-station N2 disease or consider resection for more aggressive tumors.

### Response to induction

Multimodal treatment strategies that employ induction therapy allow clinicians to gauge the biology of a tumor based on the response of the primary and nodal metastases. Multiple chemotherapy-based trials have shown improved long-term outcomes in patients with a favorable pathologic response to induction. In both the North American Intergroup 0139 trial (INT0139) and in the Radiation Therapy Oncology Group trial 0229, patients with clearance of mediastinal nodal involvement (ypN0) at resection had significantly longer OS compared to those with residual nodal disease.[27,28] Thus, the pathologic response to induction therapy presages survival. The poor outcome in patients with the residual nodal disease after induction chemotherapy led some surgeons to withhold resection in this population, whereas others proceed regardless of nodal status due to the belief that the 10% to 30% post-resection survival is better than what would be possible without resection.[3] It is unclear if the need to establish nodal clearance will be seen as a prerequisite for resection following chemo-immunotherapy. This question has new importance following induction strategies that include ICI due to the phenomenon of "pseudo-progression" or "nodal immune flair" characterized by an apparent *increase* in the size of the disease due to immune cell infiltration, as opposed to true oncologic progression. Imaging studies must be carefully interpreted, and a planned resection should not be deferred due to a radiologic increase in regional lymph nodes in response to ICI therapy.

### Pneumonectomy

The increased perioperative risk associated with pneumonectomy after induction chemotherapy, particularly with radiation therapy, has been well shown in numerous prospective trials. In the highly cited INT 0139 trial, 30% of patients in the surgical arm underwent pneumonectomy following concurrent chemotherapy and radiation with dramatically poor short- and long-term outcomes.[28] Those treated with lobectomy experienced 1% perioperative mortality, whereas patients with pneumonectomy had 27% 30-day mortality. The trial found no difference in OS between the surgical and non-surgical arm, but a post hoc analysis showed improved survival in those undergoing lobectomy when compared to a matched nonoperative group. The dramatically worse operative mortality of the pneumonectomy group was well publicized and has fueled controversy surrounding the safety of pneumonectomy following induction therapy. Importantly, in the INT 0139 trial, the majority of operations were performed by non-general thoracic surgeons, and patients with bulky N2 disease were not excluded, both are hypothesized to contribute to the high number of pneumonectomies and the associated high mortality. Numerous single-institution studies have shown acceptable perioperative morbidity and mortality for post-induction pneumonectomy when restricted to high-volume centers and when performed by general thoracic surgeons.[29] A 2012 meta-analysis including 27 trials with patients undergoing neoadjuvant therapy found 30-day perioperative mortality of 7% for patients undergoing pneumonectomy, with worse outcomes for right versus left-sided operations.[30]

More recently, in the Checkmate 816 trial, pneumonectomy was performed in 17% of patients undergoing induction nivolumab plus chemotherapy, and in 25% of those undergoing induction chemotherapy alone. Surgical outcomes for the trial were reported in 2021 and showed dramatically better short-term surgical outcomes than INT 0139. The group reported three surgery-related deaths in the trial—all in the chemotherapy arm. Grade 3 and 4 surgery-related adverse events were reported in 20%.[31] Interestingly, the trial showed regional disparity in pneumonectomy use, with higher rates of pneumonectomy and lower R1 resection rates outside North America. This suggests a potentially significant regional difference in surgical care, probably driven by a lower acceptance for pneumonectomy in North America than in Europe or Asia. It will be interesting to see if the lack of pneumonectomy-related mortality in the Check-Mate 816 and NADIM trials will change practices in North America with increased acceptance of pneumonectomy after chemo-immunotherapy.

## Neoadjuvant or Adjuvant Systemic Therapy

There are no trials directly investigating neoadjuvant versus adjuvant systemic ICI in NSCLC and each strategy has inherent advantages and disadvantages. Better treatment compliance and decreased duration of therapy are benefits of the neoadjuvant therapy regardless of the agent being used. A unique consideration for induction ICI is the presence of the large primary tumor for immune cell priming. A significant body of preclinical data shows a more intense and sustained antitumor T-cell response for neoadjuvant as opposed to adjuvant ICI.[32–34] Neoadjuvant treatment has the advantage of an intact peri-tumoral environment with intact lymphatic channels. This compares to immunotherapy delivered in the adjuvant setting, when only micro-metastatic disease is present. In addition, induction treatment gives clinicians the ability to pathologically assess the effectiveness of a drug, potentially influencing later treatment decisions. Conversely, neoadjuvant ICI therapy is not without risks; treatment-related adverse events can delay definitive surgical therapy, and some hypothesize that operations may be more difficult following the completion of neoadjuvant therapy.

Ultimately, adjuvant therapy does allow for the fastest time to surgery and thus local control, though with the risk of systemic treatment delay following surgical complications.

A head-to-head comparison of adjuvant and neoadjuvant ICI in stage III/IV resectable melanoma was reported at the European Society for Medical Oncology (ESMO) in 2022. SWOG1801 noted significant improvement in 2-year EFS with three cycles of neoadjuvant pembrolizumab compared to adjuvant pembrolizumab alone (72% vs 49%, HR 0.58: 95% CI, 0.39 to 0.87).[35] This type of trial is unlikely to be repeated in NSCLC, but the results may have a significant impact on NSCLC treatment.

## In Patients with Programmed Death-Ligand 1 <50%, Is Chemotherapy-I/O the Best Treatment?

Given the low, but real risk of immune-related adverse events, determining which patients are most likely to respond to ICI is paramount. All of the recently reported adjuvant and neoadjuvant ICI trials in NSCLC have reported outcomes stratified by level of PD-L1 expression on tumor cells, with IMpower010, CheckMate-816, and NADIM II all finding positive correlations between survival and PD-L1 expression.[13,21,22] In stage IV disease ICI therapy decisions are dictated by PD-L1 tumor expression with options for ICI alone, chemo-immunotherapy, or dual ICI based on PD-L1 expression, but those specifications do not currently exist in the adjuvant or neoadjuvant setting. For patients with intermediate levels of PD-L1 expression (1% to 49%), the benefit gained by including ICI in induction or adjuvant regimens must be balanced by the risk of adverse events. In the IMpower010 trial, 22% of patients receiving atezolizumab experienced grade 3 or 4 events, compared to 12% receiving the best supportive care. In all, 18% of patients discontinued treatment, and 12% required the use of systemic corticosteroids. In CheckMate-816, the inclusion of nivolumab did not result in an increase in adverse events; however, one still questions the benefit of a more tailored approach to increase efficacy and decrease toxicity.

## Is There Still a Role for Induction Radiotherapy?

For patients with operable stage III disease, multimodal therapy is the standard of care with induction therapy preferred over adjuvant in those with known N2 disease. Induction therapy has the benefit of early eradication of micrometastatic disease and defining tumor biology before resection.

Induction radiation therapy has been a common adjunct to chemotherapy, helping to obtain better nodal clearance before surgery, acknowledging the risk of increased operative difficulty, as well as complications such as esophagitis and pneumonitis. Inclusion of radiation in induction protocols for IIIA disease has been investigated in multiple retrospective and prospective trials, with the general finding that patients have more frequent tumor downstaging, increased rates of mediastinal nodal clearance, and increased rates of pCR, but those benefits have not translated to improved OS or DFS compared to induction chemotherapy alone.[36–39] With the introduction of neoadjuvant chemo-immunotherapy yielding increased response rates, more feasible operations, and trial data showing improved EFS, this may represent the decreased utility of radiation induction therapy. There may no longer be a need for two local modalities. In exciting work from Altorki and colleagues,[40] low-dose stereotactic body radiotherapy (SBRT) to the primary tumor alone is used with durvaulmab before resection. This chemo-free induction regime resulted in pCR rates and operative safety, which mirrored CheckMate 816, but this uses SBRT to help induce a more robust immune response and not to irradicate local or nodal disease.

## SUMMARY

Treatment of stage III lung cancer is complex and has undergone a significant paradigm shift over the last 5 years. With the expansion of ICI and targeted therapy into resectable patient populations, more patients are seeing pCRs following induction therapy, operations are being performed safely, and EFS and DFS are significantly improved. Multiple trials, including ADAURA, IMpower010, PEARLS, and CheckMate-816 have included patients with earlier-stage disease, enrolling those with stage IB-IIIA. For the IIIA population, for those with EGFR mutations, and for those with high PD-L1 scores, outcomes have been particularly encouraging. The near future holds exciting developments as the lung cancer community awaits further reports on OS as trial data mature and new controversies arise.

## CLINICS CARE POINTS

- Cure for stage IIIA non-small-cell lung cancer requires integration of local and systemic treatments, but specifics of care vary by extent of disease, patient comorbidity, and provider preferences.
- Multidisciplinary team approach is critical to the treatment of stage IIIA non-small-cell lung cancer.
- In stage IIIA non-small-cell lung cancer, biomarker testing at the time of diagnosis is essential to help guide treatment decisions.
- Although the definitions for resectability in stage IIIA may shift with the integration of novel induction therapies the need for surgical evaluation before starting treatment remains paramount.

## REFERENCES

1. Siegel RL, et al. Cancer Statistics, 2021. CA A Cancer J Clin 2021;71(1):7–33.
2. Yotsukura M, et al. Recent advances and future perspectives in adjuvant and neoadjuvant immunotherapies for lung cancer. Jpn J Clin Oncol 2020;51(1):28–36.
3. Ramnath N, et al. Treatment of Stage III Non-small Cell Lung Cancer: Diagnosis and Management of Lung Cancer, 3rd ed: American College of Chest Physicians Evidence-Based Clinical Practice Guidelines. Chest 2013;143(5):e314S–40S.
4. AJCC. AJCC cancer staging manual. 8th Ed. New York: Springer; 2016.
5. Brahmer J, et al. Nivolumab versus docetaxel in advanced squamous-cell non–small-cell lung cancer. N Engl J Med 2015;373(2):123–35.
6. Borghaei H, et al. Nivolumab versus docetaxel in advanced nonsquamous non–small-cell lung cancer. N Engl J Med 2015;373(17):1627–39.
7. Mok TSK, et al. Pembrolizumab versus chemotherapy for previously untreated, PD-L1-expressing, locally advanced or metastatic non-small-cell lung cancer (KEYNOTE-042): a randomised, open-label, controlled, phase 3 trial. Lancet 2019;393(10183):1819–30.
8. Herbst RS, et al. Pembrolizumab versus docetaxel for previously treated, PD-L1-positive, advanced non-small-cell lung cancer (KEYNOTE-010): a randomised controlled trial. Lancet 2016;387(10027):1540–50.
9. Herbst RS, et al. Atezolizumab for First-Line Treatment of PD-L1–Selected Patients with NSCLC. N Engl J Med 2020;383(14):1328–39.
10. Ramalingam SS, et al. Overall Survival with Osimertinib in Untreated, EGFR-Mutated Advanced NSCLC. N Engl J Med 2019;382(1):41–50.
11. Antonia SJ, et al. Durvalumab after Chemoradiotherapy in Stage III Non–Small-Cell Lung Cancer. N Engl J Med 2017;377(20):1919–29.

12. Antonia SJ, et al. Overall survival with durvalumab after chemoradiotherapy in stage III NSCLC. N Engl J Med 2018;379(24):2342–50.
13. Felip E, et al. Adjuvant atezolizumab after adjuvant chemotherapy in resected stage IB-IIIA non-small-cell lung cancer (IMpower010): a randomised, multicentre, open-label, phase 3 trial. Lancet 2021; 398(10308):1344–57.
14. Felip, E., Overall Survival Interim Analysis of a Phase III Study of Atezolizumab vs Best Supportive Care in Resected NSCLC, in World Conference on Lung Cancer. 2022: Vienna, Austria.
15. O'Brien M, et al. Pembrolizumab versus placebo as adjuvant therapy for completely resected stage IB-IIIA non-small-cell lung cancer (PEARLS/KEYNOTE-091): an interim analysis of a randomised, triple-blind, phase 3 trial. Lancet Oncol 2022; 23(10):1274–86.
16. Kosaka T, et al. Mutations of the epidermal growth factor receptor gene in lung cancer: biological and clinical implications. Cancer Res 2004;64(24): 8919–23.
17. Russo A, et al. Heterogeneous responses to epidermal growth factor receptor (EGFR) tyrosine kinase inhibitors (TKIs) in patients with uncommon EGFR mutations: new insights and future perspectives in this complex clinical scenario. Int J Mol Sci 2019;20(6):1431.
18. Kobayashi Y, et al. EGFR exon 18 mutations in lung cancer: molecular predictors of augmented sensitivity to afatinib or neratinib as compared with first- or third-generation TKIs. Clin Cancer Res 2015; 21(23):5305–13.
19. Wu Y-L, et al. Osimertinib in Resected EGFR-Mutated Non–Small-Cell Lung Cancer. N Engl J Med 2020;383(18):1711–23.
20. Tsuboi M, et al. LBA47 Osimertinib as adjuvant therapy in patients (pts) with resected EGFR-mutated (EGFRm) stage IB-IIIA non-small cell lung cancer (NSCLC): Updated results from ADAURA. Ann Oncol 2022;33:S1413–4.
21. Forde PM, et al. Neoadjuvant Nivolumab plus Chemotherapy in Resectable Lung Cancer. N Engl J Med 2022;386(21):1973–85.
22. Provencio-Pulla M, et al. Nivolumab + chemotherapy versus chemotherapy as neoadjuvant treatment for resectable stage IIIA NSCLC: Primary endpoint results of pathological complete response (pCR) from phase II NADIM II trial. J Clin Oncol 2022;40(16_suppl):8501.
23. Provencio M, et al. PL03.12 Progression Free Survival and Overall Survival in NADIM II Study. J Thorac Oncol 2022;17(9, Supplement):S2–3.
24. Spigel DR, et al. Five-year survival outcomes with durvalumab after chemoradiotherapy in unresectable stage III NSCLC: an update from the PACIFIC trial. J Clin Oncol 2021;39(15_suppl):8511.
25. Bryan DS, Donington JS. The role of surgery in management of locally advanced non-small cell lung cancer. Curr Treat Options Oncol 2019;20(4): 1–13.
26. Tanner NT, et al. Physician preferences for management of patients with stage IIIA NSCLC: impact of bulk of nodal disease on therapy selection. J Thorac Oncol 2012;7(2):365–9.
27. Suntharalingam M, et al. Radiation therapy oncology group protocol 02-29: a phase II trial of neoadjuvant therapy with concurrent chemotherapy and full-dose radiation therapy followed by surgical resection and consolidative therapy for locally advanced non-small cell carcinoma of the lung. Int J Radiat Oncol Biol Phys 2012;84(2):456–63.
28. Albain KS, et al. Radiotherapy plus chemotherapy with or without surgical resection for stage III non-small-cell lung cancer: a phase III randomised controlled trial. Lancet 2009;374(9687):379–86.
29. Cheung MC, et al. Impact of teaching facility status and high-volume centers on outcomes for lung cancer resection: an examination of 13,469 surgical patients. Ann Surg Oncol 2009;16(1):3–13.
30. Kim AW, et al. An analysis, systematic review, and meta-analysis of the perioperative mortality after neoadjuvant therapy and pneumonectomy for non-small cell lung cancer. J Thorac Cardiovasc Surg 2012;143(1):55–63.
31. Spicer J, et al. Surgical outcomes from the phase 3 CheckMate 816 trial: Nivolumab (NIVO) + platinum-doublet chemotherapy (chemo) vs chemo alone as neoadjuvant treatment for patients with resectable non-small cell lung cancer (NSCLC). J Clin Oncol 2021;39(15_suppl):8503.
32. Liu J, et al. Improved Efficacy of Neoadjuvant Compared to Adjuvant Immunotherapy to Eradicate Metastatic Disease. Cancer Discov 2016;6(12): 1382–99.
33. Blank CU, et al. Neoadjuvant versus adjuvant ipilimumab plus nivolumab in macroscopic stage III melanoma. Nat Med 2018;24(11):1655–61.
34. Donington JS. Neoadjuvant Immunotherapy for Resectable Non-small Cell Lung Cancer: Exciting New Horizon in Early-Stage Lung Cancer Care. Ann Surg Oncol 2022;29(9):5344–6.
35. Patel S, et al. LBA6 Neoadjuvant versus adjuvant pembrolizumab for resected stage III-IV melanoma (SWOG S1801). Ann Oncol 2022;33:S1408.
36. Pless M, et al. Induction chemoradiation in stage IIIA/N2 non-small-cell lung cancer: a phase 3 randomised trial. Lancet 2015;386(9998):1049–56.
37. Katakami N, et al. A phase 3 study of induction treatment with concurrent chemoradiotherapy versus chemotherapy before surgery in patients with pathologically confirmed N2 stage IIIA nonsmall cell lung cancer (WJTOG9903). Cancer 2012;118(24): 6126–35.

38. Chen Y, et al. Comparing the benefits of chemora-diotherapy and chemotherapy for resectable stage III A/N2 non-small cell lung cancer: a meta-analysis. World J Surg Oncol 2018;16(1):8.

39. Higgins K, et al. Preoperative chemotherapy versus preoperative chemoradiotherapy for stage III (N2) non-small-cell lung cancer. Int J Radiat Oncol Biol Phys 2009;75(5):1462–7.

40. Altorki NK, et al. Neoadjuvant durvalumab with or without stereotactic body radiotherapy in patients with early-stage non-small-cell lung cancer: a single-centre, randomised phase 2 trial. Lancet Oncol 2021;22(6):824–35.

# Neoadjuvant Strategies for Esophageal Cancer
## Role of Immunotherapy and Positron emission tomography (PET)-Guided Strategies

Carly C. Barron, MD, MSc[a,b,1], Xin Wang, MD, PhD[a,b,1], Elena Elimova, MD, MSc[b,*]

## KEYWORDS

- Esophageal cancer • Adenocarcinoma • Squamous cell carcinoma • Neoadjuvant treatment
- Immunotherapy • FDG-PET • Biomarkers

## KEY POINTS

- Multimodal management with chemotherapy with or without radiation prior to surgery is the standard of care for locally advanced esophageal cancer.
- Adjuvant nivolumab for patients with residual disease following trimodality therapy improves disease-free survival.
- Phase II evidence suggests treatment with neoadjuvant immune checkpoint inhibitors improves pathological complete response, multiple phase III trials are ongoing.
- FDG-PET, when used during neoadjuvant treatment, has prognostic and predictive value, although the optimal parameters to differentiate responders and non-responders require further study.
- Use of biomarkers including MSI and CPS remains crucial for selecting patients most likely to benefit from addition of immunotherapy to perioperative management.

## BACKGROUND

Esophageal cancer is the eighth most common cancer worldwide, and despite advances in detection and management, continues to have a high mortality rate.[1] More than half of patients present with advanced or metastatic disease with median survival of less than 1 year.[2] In the locally advanced setting, esophagectomy has been the mainstay of treatment but nearly half of the patients have locoregional or distant recurrence with surgery alone. Multimodal management with chemotherapy with or without radiation before surgery improves disease-free and overall survival (OS).[3,4]

To further improve outcomes for these patients, important questions surrounding neoadjuvant and adjuvant strategies for patients with locally advanced esophageal cancer have been posed. Given the benefit of treatment with immune checkpoint inhibitors (ICIs) seen for patients with metastatic esophageal cancer,[5] the role of immunotherapy has been explored before and after

[a] Medical Oncology Training Program, OPG 7-7W259, University of Toronto, Toronto, Ontario, M5G 2M9, Canada; [b] Division of Medical Oncology, Princess Margaret Cancer Centre, OPG 7-715, 610 University Avenue, Toronto, Ontario M5G 2M9, Canada

[1] These authors contributed equally to this work.

* Corresponding author. Princess Margaret Cancer Centre, OPG 7-715, 610 University Avenue, Toronto, Ontario M5G 2M9, Canada.

E-mail address: Elena.elimova@uhn.ca

Twitter: @carlycbarron (C.C.B.); @KevinXinWang (X.W.)

Thorac Surg Clin 33 (2023) 197–208

https://doi.org/10.1016/j.thorsurg.2023.01.009

surgery in the curative setting. In addition, efforts to individualize treatment have led to the inclusion of PET imaging in the neoadjuvant setting to guide treatment decisions and to determine its utility as a biomarker.[6]

In this article, we provide an overview of the current perioperative management of locally advanced esophageal cancer, with an emphasis on incorporating immunotherapy in the adjuvant setting and recent advances exploring the role of ICIs and PET in guiding neoadjuvant management.

## DIFFERENCES IN HISTOLOGICAL SUBTYPES

There are important differences between the adenocarcinoma (AC) and squamous cell carcinoma (SCC) histological subtypes of esophageal cancer with respect to risk factors, clinical behavior, and recurrence patterns. The incidence of esophageal SCC has decreased in Western countries in part due to decreased smoking and alcohol use; however, the incidence of AC has reciprocally increased with the rise in gastroesophageal reflux disease and body mass index.[7] Worldwide, the incidence of SCC remains high, particularly in Eastern Asia and Africa.[8] SCCs have a higher perioperative mortality than ACs despite being diagnosed at an earlier age on average.[9] In terms of recurrence, ACs tend to recur distantly, whereas SCCs have higher rates of muscle or nodal recurrence.[10] In recent years, the molecular differences between SCC and AC have become better understood. The Cancer Genome Atlas project performed a comprehensive molecular analysis and found that esophageal SCCs resembled squamous carcinomas of other organs, such as head and neck cancers.[11] On the contrary, esophageal AC more resembled the chromosomally unstable variant of gastric AC, suggesting these cancers may be a single disease entity. Furthermore, these differences are also reflected in the varying tumor microenvironment between the subtypes and the response to targeted therapies and immunotherapy.[12] Esophageal SCC has generally been grouped with esophageal AC in clinical trials. However, given the etiological, biological, and clinical differences, future trials should separate these distinct histologies.

## MANAGEMENT OF LOCALLY ADVANCED ESOPHAGEAL CARCINOMA

The treatment of locally advanced SCC and AC requires a multidisciplinary discussion and approach. The current standard of care for patients with an adequate performance status and resectable disease is chemoradiation therapy (CRT) followed by surgery and adjuvant nivolumab in the absence of a complete pathological response (pCR). In those with unresectable disease, or who decline surgery, definitive CRT can be considered.

### Perioperative Chemotherapy

Historically, perioperative chemotherapy showed modest survival benefits. This was first shown in the OEO2 trial by the Medical Research Council, which compared preoperative cisplatin and 5FU with surgery alone in both SCC and AC, offering a survival benefit of 5-year OS 23% versus 17%, respectively (OEO2). The pivotal Medical Research Council Adjuvant Gastric Infusional Chemotherapy (MAGIC) trial included mainly AC and showed a triplet combination of epirubicin, cisplatin, and 5-FU (ECF) was superior to surgery alone with 5-year OS 36% versus 23%, respectively (MAGIC). More recently, the FLOT4 trial, which compared EGJ and gastric AC using a triplet chemotherapy FLOT (docetaxel, oxaliplatin, leucovorin, and 5FU) showed superiority over an anthracycline-based triplet chemotherapy, with 3-year OS 57% versus 48%, respectively, HR 0.77, $P = .004$ (FLOT4).[4] These regimens are summarized in **Table 1**.

### Concurrent Chemoradiation

Multiple studies have shown a survival benefit using preoperative concurrent chemoradiotherapy over surgery alone. These trials included patients with both AC and SCC. The ChemoRadiotherapy for Oesophageal cancer followed by Surgery Study (CROSS) trial was a randomized phase III study in which patients with resectable esophageal cancer were assigned to surgery alone or CRT with weekly carboplatin and paclitaxel for 5 weeks followed by surgery. The majority of patients in this study had AC (75%), whereas 23% had squamous-cell carcinoma. The pCR rate in patients who underwent CRT was 29%, with patients with SCC having a significantly higher rate than those with AC at 49%. Updated data at 10 years show a stable effect on OS at 38% in the CRT group and 25% in the surgery alone group with an absolute benefit of 13%.[13] Another neoadjuvant phase III trial, CALGB 9781, randomized patients to preoperative fluorouracil and cisplatin plus radiation versus surgery alone.[14] The CRT group had a 40% pCR rate and 5-year OS rates were 39% versus 16% in the surgery-alone group. FOLFOX plus radiation is another acceptable preoperative regimen as evaluated in the SWOG phase II trial.[15] The pCR rate was similar at 28% with a 3-year OS of 45%.

**Table 1**
Perioperative chemotherapy and chemoradiation in the pre-immunotherapy era

| Reference | Tumor Location | N | SCC/AC% | Comparison | Outcome | Surgical Outcome |
|---|---|---|---|---|---|---|
| RTOG 8911/Intergroup 0113 | Esophagus, EGJ | 440 | 47/53 | Surgery vs preoperative cisplatin + 5FU | Median OS 16.1 m vs 14.9 m ($P$ = .53), 2-y OS 26% vs 23% ($P$ = .65) | R0 resection rate 59% vs 63% |
| JCOG 9907 | Esophagus | 330 | 100/0 | Postoperative cisplatin + 5FU vs preoperative cisplatin + 5FU | 5-y OS 42% vs 55% ($P$ = .04) | R0 resection rate 91% vs 96% ($P$ = .04) |
| OEO2 | Esophagus, EGJ | 802 | 31/66 | Surgery vs preoperative cisplatin + 5FU | 5-y OS 17% vs 23% ($P$ = .004) | R0 resection rate 54% vs 60% |
| MAGIC | Lower esophagus, EGJ, stomach | 503 | 0/100 | Surgery vs perioperative ECF | 5-y OS 23% vs 36% (.009) | R0 resection rate 70% vs 79% ($P$ = .03) |
| CROSS | Esophagus, EGJ | 368 | 25/75 | Surgery vs preoperative carboplatin + paclitaxel + CRT | 5-y OS 34% vs 47% ($P$ = .003) | R0 resection rate 69% vs 92% ($P$ < .001) |
| ACCORD07 | Lower esophagus, EGJ, stomach | 224 | 0/100 | Surgery vs perioperative cisplatin + 5FU | 5-y OS 24% vs 38% ($P$ = .02) | R0 resection rate 74% vs 84% ($P$ = .04) |
| FLOT4-AIO | EGJ, stomach | 716 | 0/100 | Perioperative ECF/ECX vs perioperative FLOT | 5-y OS 36% vs 45%, HR 0.77 ($P$ = .012) | R0 resection rate 78% vs 85% ($P$ = .0162) |

Adapted from Mayanagi S, Irino T, Kawakubo H, Kitagawa Y. Neoadjuvant treatment strategy for locally advanced thoracic esophageal cancer. Ann Gastroenterol Surg. 2019;3(3):269-275.

Only one study, the NEOCRTEC5010 trial, has looked exclusively at the benefit of neoadjuvant CRT in SCC.[16] Previous randomized controlled trials had shown inconsistent benefits in OS with combined modality treatment over surgery alone in SCC based on a small number of patients. The objective of the NEOCRTEC5010 trial was to determine if neoadjuvant CRT plus surgery improved OS over surgery alone. The chemotherapy regimen used was cisplatin and vinorelbine. The results showed that the pCR rate was 43.2% in the CRT group with a median OS of 100 months, which was improved compared with 66.5 months in the surgery arm (hazard ratio [HR] 0.71, 95% confidence interval [CI] 0.53 to 0.96, $P = .025$).

Given SCC trended toward a better response than AC in the pivotal CROSS trial, the optimal treatment of AC was actively investigated. The landmark FLOT4-AIO trial as discussed above definitively showed that FLOT was superior to ECF/ECX with an HR of 0.77 leading to a median OS of 50 months versus 35 months.[4] The more recent Neo-AEGIS trial attempted to address whether neoadjuvant CRT with CROSS regimen can outperform optimum perioperative chemotherapy consisting of MAGIC regimen and later FLOT.[17] This randomized trial enrolled 377 patients with AEG AC to CROSS of chemotherapy (MAGIC, later amended to FLOT following the results of FLOT4-AIO). This trial showed a similar 3-year estimated survival probability of 56% (95% CI 47.64) with CROSS and 57% (95% CI 48.65) with MAGIC/FLOT, with an HR 1.02. Based on futility, this trial has closed recruitment. Looking closely at the secondary endpoints, more patients on CROSS had an R0 resection (95% vs 82%) and pathologic complete response (16% vs 5%).

Two ongoing phase III clinical trials, ESOPEC and POWERRANGER, which all enrolled esophageal and EGJ AC, will shed further light on this clinical quagmire. Like Neo-AEGIS, ESOPEC is a phase III trial comparing perioperative FLOT to neoadjuvant CROSS to determine which protocol is superior; the primary endpoint will be OS.[18] POWERRANGER has a similar design to ESOPEC, but also includes ECF/ECX as a possible comparator arm, with a primary outcome of treatment response (NCT01404156).

### Definitive Chemoradiation

Given the sensitivity of SCC to CRT, the necessity of surgery for patients with tumors of this histological subtype has been questioned. A randomized trial by Stahl and colleagues[19] assigned patients with locally advanced esophageal SCC to induction chemotherapy followed by CRT then surgery, or induction chemotherapy followed by definitive CRT. The group that underwent surgery had an improved local progression-free survival (HR 2.1, 95% CI 1.3 to 3.5, $P = .003$); however, OS did not significantly differ between the two groups. A lack of difference in survival was also shown in the FFCD 9102 trial in which patients with esophageal SCC who had a response to induction CRT were randomized to continue this or undergo surgery.[20] Despite these findings, the National Comprehensive Cancer Network (NCCN) guidelines recommend the inclusion of surgery rather than definitive CRT alone given the efficacy and safety seen in the CROSS trial. For patients who are not fit for surgery CRT is an acceptable alternative.

### Adjuvant Nivolumab

The Checkmate 577 trial established adjuvant nivolumab as the standard of care for patients with esophageal cancer who previously received neoadjuvant CRT following complete resection with residual pathologic disease.[21] Of the patients included in the study, 29% had SCC. Disease-free survival (DFS) was significantly longer in patients who had received 1 year of adjuvant nivolumab compared with those that received placebo (median DFS 22.4 vs 11 m, HR 0.69, 96.4% CI 0.56 to 0.86, $P < .001$). In a prespecified post hoc analysis of patients with SCC, the absolute benefit was larger with a median DFS of 29.7 months in the nivolumab group compared with 11 months in the placebo group (HR 0.61, 95% CI 0.42 to 0.88). Additional analyses suggest that the survival benefit may be driven by programmed death-ligand 1 (PD-L1) expression, as patients with combined positive score (CPS) greater than 5 had a significantly longer median DFS of 29.4 months (HR 0.62 95%CI 0.46 to 0.83), whereas those with CPS less than 5 showed only a marginal trend toward improved DFS (HR 0.89, 95% CI 0.65 to 1.22). This is similar to the improved response in patients with CPS greater than 5 that was seen with nivolumab in the metastatic setting in gastric cancers in Checkmate 649.[22] The role of PD-L1 in predicting response to checkpoint inhibitors in the adjuvant setting remains to further elucidated.

In Checkmate 577, distant metastasis-free survival was also improved in the nivolumab group at a median of 28.3 m compared with 17.6 m (HR 0.74, 95% CI 0.60 to 0.92). Grade 3 or 4 adverse events related to the study treatment were similar in each group (13% vs 6%) and the most common toxicities related to nivolumab included fatigue, diarrhea, pruritus, and rash. Based on the results of this study the US Food and Drug Administration has approved adjuvant nivolumab for patients who meet Checkmate 577 inclusion criteria, and this regimen has been endorsed by NCCN and updated American Society of Clinical Oncology (ASCO) guidelines.[23]

### Role of Immunotherapy

**Rationale for neoadjuvant checkpoint blockade**
Several ongoing studies are exploring whether the addition of ICIs in the neoadjuvant management of esophageal cancers can improve patient outcomes. Using immunotherapy in the neoadjuvant setting may offer several advantages. Evidence from the metastatic setting has shown improved response rates and survival when immunotherapy is added to chemotherapy compared with chemotherapy alone. The KEYNOTE 590 trial randomized patients with unresectable or metastatic esophageal cancer to 5-fluorouracil and cisplatin plus pembrolizumab or placebo.[5] Patients in the chemotherapy and immunotherapy group had a response rate of 45% versus 29.3% in the chemotherapy plus placebo group. In patients with tumors of squamous histology, the OS was improved with addition of pembrolizumab at a median of 12.6 months versus 9.8 months (HR 0.72 95% CI 0.60 to 0.88, $P = .0006$). Treatment-related adverse events were similar in the two groups at 72% and 68% respectively. Therefore, given that the addition of immunotherapy is well-tolerated and may downstage disease and allow for R0 resection, this represents an attractive strategy.

The improvement in DFS in the aforementioned Checkmate 577 study suggests that adjuvant nivolumab may eliminate micrometastatic disease. Indeed, an improvement in DFS from adjuvant immunotherapy has been shown in several other cancer types including melanoma, lung, and bladder.[24–26] Using immunotherapy neoadjuvantly to try to eradicate micrometastatic disease, instead of adjuvantly, is of specific interest in esophageal cancer due to the morbidity of the surgery. Approximately 50% of patients are not fit to complete adjuvant therapy because of poor nutrition after surgery and toxicities. Administering immunotherapy before surgery could increase compliance and avoid delays due to surgical complications.

It has been suggested that using a neoadjuvant strategy may produce a more robust immune response due to the presence of multiple antigens from the tumor.[27] In addition, the immune mediating effects of radiation and chemotherapy may enhance the efficacy of ICIs. Both chemotherapy and radiation have been shown to upregulate the expression of PD-L1 in the tumor immune microenvironment.[28,29] Whether there is synergy between CRT and immunotherapy leading to a more durable response remains to be determined (**Table 2**).

### Evidence

Early results from phase I and II trials in esophageal SCC suggest that neoadjuvant checkpoint blockade is safe and increases pCR rates (see **Table 2**). Preoperative Anti-PD-1 Antibody combined with Chemoradiotherapy for Locally Advanced Squmous Cell Carcinoma of Esophageus-2 (PALACE-2) was a single-arm trial of neoadjuvant pembrolizumab combined with CRT for locally advanced ESCC.[30] Included patients had T2-T4a disease without lymph node involvement or evidence of metastasis and an Eastern Cooperative Oncology Group (ECOG) performance status of 0 to 1. The treatment regimen consisted of carboplatin and paclitaxel weekly for 5 weeks, pembrolizumab given on days 1 and 22, and 41.4 Gy of radiation delivered in 23 fractions. Twenty patients were enrolled of which only one was female. Eighteen patients underwent surgery as one patient had disease progression and one patient died from an esophageal hemorrhage while awaiting surgery. The pCR rate in ten patients at 56% was higher than the 49% seen in the SCC group of CROSS. At a median follow-up of 6.6 months all patients who underwent resection were free of disease recurrence. The rate of grade 3 or greater AEs was 65% consisting mostly of hematological AEs (leukopenia, neutropenia, lymphopenia) and one patient with esophageal hemorrhage. Although this study had a small sample size without randomization, the high rate of pCR and comparable safety profile to the CROSS study warrants further investigation. The PALACE-2 phase II multicenter study is currently underway.

Neoadjuvant Pembrolizumab and Chemotherapy in Resectable Esophageal Cancer: An Open-Label, Single-Arm Study (PEN-ICE) was an open-label single-arm study that looked at the role of neoadjuvant pembrolizumab compared with platinum-based chemotherapy alone for three cycles before surgery.[31] The chemotherapy regimens were based on physicians choice and all of them contained docetaxel or nab-paclitaxel with nedaplatin. Eighteen patients were enrolled of which 13 underwent resection; 4 patients declined surgery after symptomatic relief from neoadjuvant therapy and 1 patient had disease progression and was given definitive CRT. Postoperative pathology showed that 46% of patients had a pCR. Five patients (28%) experienced grade 3/4 treat-related AEs with one patient with a history of pulmonary

**Table 2**
Ongoing trials using checkpoint inhibitors in the curative setting in esophageal cancer

| Trial | Treatment Approach | Phase | Population | Investigational Arm | Control | Primary Outcome |
|---|---|---|---|---|---|---|
| PALACE-2 | Neoadjuvant | II | Esophageal SCC | Preoperative CRT (carboplatin, paclitaxel) + pembrolizumab | n/a | pCR |
| KEYNOTE 975 | Definitive | III | Esophageal/GEJ SCC, adenocarcinoma | CRT (5-FU/Platinum or FOLFOX) + Pembrolizumab | CRT (5-FU/Platinum or FOLFOX) + Placebo | OS EFS |
| SKYSCRAPER-07 | Definitive | III | Esophageal SCC | Atezolizumab + tiragolumab after definitive CRT | Atezolizumab + placebo after definitive CRT | PFS OS |
| KEYNOTE 585 | Perioperative | III | Gastric/GEJ adenocarcinoma | Perioperative 5-FU/cisplatin or capecitabine + Pembrolizumab | Perioperative 5-FU/cisplatin or capecitabine + Placebo | EFS pCR OS AE |
| MATTERHORN | Perioperative | III | Gastric/GEJ adenocarcinoma | Perioperative FLOT + durvalumab | Perioperative FLOT + placebo | EFS |
| VESTIGE | Adjuvant | II | Gastric/Esophageal adenocarcinoma | Adjuvant nivolumab and ipilimumab | Continue preoperative chemotherapy | DFS |
| DANTE | Perioperative | II | Gastric/GEJ adenocarcinoma | Perioperative FLOT + atezolizumab | Perioperative FLOT | DFS/PFS |

fibrosis that developed pneumonitis and pneumonia post-resection and died. This study highlights the importance of patient selection when considering neoadjuvant immunotherapy and may play a role for patients with contraindications to radiation. The results should be confirmed with randomized evidence.

For patients who are unable to undergo resection, immunotherapy in addition to definitive CRT may improve outcomes in the first-line setting. Keynote 975 is a double blind, phase III randomized placebo-controlled trial in which patients are assigned to receive definitive CRT with either placebo or pembrolizumab 200 mg every 3 weeks for 8 cycles followed by 400 mg every 6 weeks for 5 cycles.[32] The accepted CRT regimens will include cisplatin and 5-FU with 50 or 60 Gy of radiation, or FOLFOX with 50 Gy radiation. Randomization will be stratified by PD-L1 status, radiation dose, geographic region, and histology. The included patients are those with locally advanced unresectable esophageal squamous cell carcinoma (ESCC), gastroesophageal junction (GEJ) cancer, esophageal adenocarcinoma (EAC), or cervical or upper thoracic esophageal carcinoma with supraclavicular lymph node metastases only. The dual-primary endpoints are OS and event-free survival (EFS) per blinded independent central review or biopsy in all patients, in patients with ESCC, and in patients with tumor PD-L1 expression of CPS $\geq$10. The study is recruiting and the anticipated completion is in 2026. The results of this study will be important for the proportion of patients with locally advanced diseases who are unable to undergo surgery for which the treatment options are limited and recurrence is high.

The phase III SKYSCRAPER-07 study aimed to enhance the efficacy of anti-PD-L1 blockade with the addition of an anti-T cell immunoreceptor with immunoglobulin and ITIM domain (TIGIT) agent.[33] The TIGIT pathway is involved in the regulation of T cell- and natural killer cell-mediated tumor recognition, and combined with PD-1/PD-L1 blockade may lead to enhanced T-cell function and expansion.[34] This strategy was tested in patients with advanced non-small-cell lung cancer in the phase II CITYSCAPE trial and was shown to increase objective response rate (ORR) and progression-free survival (PFS) with an acceptable safety profile.[35] The SKYSCRAPER-07 study will randomize patients with unresectable esophageal SCC without progressive disease after platinum-based definitive CRT to the anti-TIGIT antibody tiragolumab plus atezolizumab, placebo plus atezolizumab or double placebo for up to 17 cycles. The co-primary endpoints are investigator-assessed PFS and OS.

Given the results of Checkmate 577, several large phase III trials will investigate whether the addition of immunotherapy to perioperative chemotherapy will provide similar benefits in patients with gastric and GEJ AC. The phase IIb DANTE study with recruitment largely in Germany and Switzerland will explore whether the addition of atezolizumab to perioperative FLOT will improve its primary outcome of DFS/PFS.[36] 295 patients with resectable AC of the stomach and GEJ ($\geq$cT2 and/or N+) were randomized. The preliminary results were recently presented at ASCO 2022 which showed similar tolerability, but more pathological regression favoring atezolizumab, with pT0 rates of 23% versus 15%, pN0 rates of 68% versus 54% in the atezolizumab and FLOT arms, respectively.

The international MATTERHORN trial, which is recruiting at 175 institutions, will study the combination of durvalumab with FLOT versus FLOT alone.[37] This is a phase III double-blind, randomized trial evaluating the efficacy and safety of neoadjuvant-adjuvant durvalumab or placebo with FLOT followed by adjuvant durvalumab or placebo in patients with resectable gastric and GEJ cancers. This trial aims to recruit 900 patients and is awaiting readout. The primary endpoint is EFS and the secondary endpoint will explore OS and pCR. Dual checkpoint blockade using the combination nivolumab and ipilimumab will be studied in the EA2174 randomized phase II/III trial, which is actively recruiting.[38] This trial will enroll esophageal and GEJ AC and randomize patients to preoperative CRT (carboplatin AUC 2 IV and paclitaxel 50 mg/m2 IV), both weekly x 5 during concurrent radiation (50.4 Gy) versus the addition of nivolumab alone or in combination with ipilimumab. Patients with no postoperative disease receive nivolumab 240 mg IV every 2 weeks for 12 cycles either with or without ipilimumab 1 mg/kg IV every 6 weeks for 4 cycles. The primary neoadjuvant endpoint is pCR rate and the primary adjuvant endpoint is DFS. Finally, in a largely Asian population, ATTRACTION-05, will explore whether the addition of nivolumab in combination with adjuvant S-1 or CAPOX chemotherapy will improve the primary endpoint of RFS.[39] This is a randomized phase III trial of in the adjuvant setting for patients with pathologic stage III gastric and GEJ cancer with treatment continued for up to 1 year. The preliminary results of these perioperative immunotherapy trials are anticipated within the next few years.

### Microsatellite Instability-High Tumors

Although microsatellite instability is common in gastric cancer, the proportion of MSI-H esophageal cancer is only about 1%.[40] Multiple studies have shown that patients with GEJ and gastric cancers with an MSI-H phenotype have a better prognosis regardless of disease stage.[41] The benefit of perioperative chemotherapy in this patient population has been questioned and a large meta-analysis failed to show an improvement in DFS when chemotherapy was added over surgery alone.[42] The phase II GERCOR NEONIPIGA evaluated whether immunotherapy has efficacy in the perioperative setting for patients with localized gastroesophageal AC.[43] Patients who were treated with neo-adjuvant nivolumab and ipilimumab followed by adjuvant nivolumab had a pCR of 59%. These results were based on just 32 patients and data from a larger sample with information about survival outcomes are pending. Until additional information is available regarding patient selection, and benefit of ICIs, the management of patients with locally advanced MSI-H tumors should involve a multidisciplinary discussion.

## POSITRON EMISSION TOMOGRAPHY (PET)-DIRECTED THERAPY
### Staging and Detection of Occult Metastatic Disease

Fluorodeoxyglucose (FDG) PET is part of the standard staging of esophageal cancer. In patients who do not have any evidence of distant metastases after contrast-enhanced CT, FDG-PET is more sensitive to detect occult metastatic disease. A prospective study showed that the addition of FDG-PET detected additional sites of disease in 41% of patients and resulted in significant changes in management in 38% of patients.[44] In a multicenter prospective cohort study of patients with potentially resectable esophageal cancer, FDG-PET led to changes in stage for 24% of patients, the majority (21.8%) were upstaged.[45]

For early-stage tumors, FDG-PET has a limited role in determining the depth of tumor invasion and has a high rate of false-positive findings.[46] In addition, it has a low sensitivity for detecting locoregional nodal involvement as the metabolic activity from the primary tumor can affect uptake into the surrounding nodes.[46,47] Therefore, the main diagnostic benefit of FDG-PET is for staging cM disease and determining which patients may be appropriate for resection.

### Assessment of Response to Neoadjuvant Treatment

As discussed above, neoadjuvant multimodality strategies lead to pathological downstaging, increase in R0 resection rates, and a decrease in recurrent disease. Despite this, the most common

reason for treatment failure is distant recurrence. Given the utility and adoption of FDG-PET for the initial staging and detection of recurrence, it has been hypothesized that FDG-PET may have a role in differentiating responders versus nonresponders during neoadjuvant treatment. Identification of patients with poor response to neoadjuvant CRT can avoid unnecessary treatment-related toxicity. A systematic review of 13 studies, largely of retrospective cohorts, showed modest evidence with 8 studies showing a correlation between the PET parameter and pathological response or the studied clinical outcome.[48] Early prospective studies suggested that PET imaging may differentiate responding and nonresponding tumors early on in the course of therapy and in doing so can offer prognostic information.[49,50]

Several recent prospective trials have explored the role of FDG-PET in predicting histopathological response and survival. The MUNICON-1 and 2 prospective trials attempted to answer this question. In MUNICON-1, 119 patients with locally advanced AC of AEG type 1 or 2 were enrolled and treated with chemotherapy, 49% of patients had a metabolic response at week 2, which was defined by a decrease of 35% or more in tumor glucose SUV.[51] 58% of patients in the metabolic responders had a major histological remission, defined as less than 10% residual tumor at resection. However, no histological response was noted in the metabolic nonresponders. Median OS was 25.8 months in the nonresponders and was not reached in the responders, with an HR 2.13, CI 1.14 to 3.99, $P = .015$.

The follow-up MUNICON-2 trial attempted to salvage metabolic nonresponders with neoadjuvant radiochemotherapy.[52] Of 23 metabolic nonresponders, 6 subsequently had histologic remission. However, the primary endpoint of R0 resection rate was not met. The use of PET to identify nonresponders may potentially save time and reduce unnecessary side effects and costs.

In the AGITG DOCTOR phase II study, 124 patients with resectable esophageal AC received induction cisplatin and 5-fluorouracil (CF) and were assessed by PET at day 15.[53] Patients with an early metabolic response, which is defined by a [SUV]max of 35% reduction from baseline to day 15 received an additional cycle of chemotherapy. Nonresponders were randomized 1:1 to either two cycles of CF and docetaxel (DCF) or DCF plus 45 Gray radiotherapy, followed by esophagectomy. The primary endpoint was a major histological response (<10% residual tumor) in the esophagectomy specimen. Secondary endpoints were OS, PFS, and locoregional recurrence. This study showed that a major histological response was achieved in 7% of patients with an early metabolic response by PET. Looking at survival at 60 months, 53% were alive if they achieved early metabolic response versus 31% and 46% for nonresponders that were randomized to additional treatment. This study showed that early metabolic response is associated with favorable OS, PFS, and low local-regional recurrence.[54]

More recently, the CALGB 80803 trial used FDG-PET to tailor therapy based on whether patients responded to upfront chemotherapy.[55] In total, 241 patients were randomized to FOLFOX or carboplatin-paclitaxel, and repeat FDG-PET was performed after 6 weeks of induction therapy. Nonresponders switched to the alternate chemotherapy during CRT (50.4 Gy/28 fractions). Interestingly, with this approach, the pCR rates in the initial nonresponders cohort were around 20%. Median OS was 48.8 months in the PET responders and 27.4 months in the nonresponders, again pointing to worse biology in the nonresponders group.

The precise PET parameter that has the best predictive value is hotly debated and an area of ongoing research. Several traditional PET parameters have been studied to correlate with pathological response. These include the maximum and mean standardized uptake value (SUVmax and SUVmean), metabolic tumor volume (MTV), and total lesion glycolysis (TLG).[56] One study of 31 patients with resectable esophageal SCC or AC were followed prospectively with PET during treatment with trimodality therapy and showed that baseline TLG and post-chemoradiotherapy TLG were associated with OS.[57] More recently, radiomic signatures are being actively developed for more robust predictions. Simoni and colleagues,[58] in a retrospective analysis, investigated multiple traditional PET parameters and identified several radiomic features as well as tumor regression grade being correlated with pathologic response. Further studies will be needed to develop more reliable predictive models and be tested in prospective randomized trials. Furthermore, whether these strategies hold true in the era of immunotherapy remains largely unknown.

## SUMMARY AND FUTURE DIRECTIONS

Significant progress has been made in the management of locally advanced esophageal cancer in recent years. Adjuvant nivolumab represents a new standard of care for patients with residual disease following trimodality therapy, especially in patients with SCC. There is early-phase evidence that treatment with neoadjuvant ICIs may improve pCR and DFS; however, larger randomized studies

are needed to confirm this. The optimal combination of chemoimmunotherapy will be critical to determine the most efficacious regimen. With changes in the neoadjuvant space moving forwards, physicians must give careful consideration to applying evidence to individual patients and personalizing management. Given that patients with PD-L1 high tumors have shown the greatest survival benefit from ICIs, biomarker selection remains critical, and all patients should have MSI and CPS testing at diagnosis. However, there remain significant challenges in selecting more reliable predictive biomarkers; as such more correlative studies are necessary. The expanding role of PET may help guide decisions and tailor neoadjuvant therapy. With the implementation of artificial intelligence and machine learning, radiomics signatures may be the future in finding imaging-based predictive biomarkers. Multidisciplinary collaboration from surgery, radiation, and medical oncology in encouraging patient participation in clinical trials, and planning and executing future studies, will continue to drive the field forwards.

## CLINICS CARE POINTS

- In patients newly diagnosed with re-sectable esophageal cancer, MSI and CPS status should be reflexively done on all patients due to its prognostic and/or predictive value.
- FDG-PET is widely used in staging, it's utility in neoadjuvant treatment is exploratory.

## DISCLOSURE

Dr E. Elimova has disclosed participating in research for Bristol-Myers Squibb and Zymeworks; serving on a data safety monitoring board for Zymeworks; serving as an advisory board member and as a consultant for Zymeworks, Bristol Myers Squibb, Adaptimmune Therapeutics, and BeiGene; and having a spouse employed by Merck. The remaining authors have disclosed that they have not received any financial consideration from any person or organization to support this work.

## REFERENCES

1. Sung H, Ferlay J, Siegel RL, et al. Global Cancer Statistics 2020: GLOBOCAN estimates of incidence and mortality worldwide for 36 cancers in 185 countries. CA A Cancer J Clin 2021;71(3):209–49.
2. Wang X, Espin-Garcia O, Jiang DM, et al. Impact of sites of metastatic dissemination on survival in

advanced gastroesophageal adenocarcinoma. Oncology 2022;100(8):439–48.

3. Shapiro J, van Lanschot JJB, Hulshof MCCM, et al. Neoadjuvant chemoradiotherapy plus surgery versus surgery alone for oesophageal or junctional cancer (CROSS): long-term results of a randomised controlled trial. Lancet Oncol 2015;16(9):1090–8.

4. Al-Batran S-E, Homann N, Pauligk C, et al. Perioperative chemotherapy with fluorouracil plus leucovorin, oxaliplatin, and docetaxel versus fluorouracil or capecitabine plus cisplatin and epirubicin for locally advanced, resectable gastric or gastro-oesophageal junction adenocarcinoma (FLOT4): a ra. Lancet 2019;393(10184):1948–57.

5. Sun JM, Shen L, Shah MA, et al. Pembrolizumab plus chemotherapy versus chemotherapy alone for first-line treatment of advanced oesophageal cancer (KEYNOTE-590): a randomised, placebo-controlled, phase 3 study. Lancet 2021;398(10302):759–71.

6. de Geus-Oei LF, Slingerland M. PET-guided treatment algorithms in oesophageal cancer: the promise of the near future. J Thorac Dis 2017;9(9):2736–9.

7. Thrift AP. The epidemic of oesophageal carcinoma: where are we now? Cancer Epidemiol 2016;41:88–95.

8. Morgan E, Soerjomataram I, Rumgay H, et al. the global landscape of esophageal squamous cell carcinoma and esophageal adenocarcinoma incidence and mortality in 2020 and projections to 2040: new estimates from GLOBOCAN 2020. Gastroenterology 2022;163(3):649–58.e2.

9. Alexandrou A, Davis PA, Law S, et al. Squamous cell carcinoma and adenocarcinoma of the lower third of the esophagus and gastric cardia: similarities and differences. Dis Esophagus 2002;15(4):290–5.

10. Rustgi A, El-Serag HB. Esophageal carcinoma. N Engl J Med 2015;372(15):1472–3.

11. Kim J, Bowlby R, Mungall AJ, et al. Integrated genomic characterization of oesophageal carcinoma. Nature 2017;541(7636):169–74.

12. Davern M, Donlon NE, Power R, et al. The tumour immune microenvironment in oesophageal cancer. Br J Cancer 2021;125(4):479–94.

13. Eyck BM, van Lanschot JJB, Hulshof MCCM, et al. Ten-year outcome of neoadjuvant chemoradiotherapy plus surgery for esophageal cancer: The Randomized Controlled CROSS Trial. J Clin Oncol 2021;39(18):1995–2004.

14. Tepper J, Krasna MJ, Niedzwiecki D, et al. Phase III trial of trimodality therapy with cisplatin, fluorouracil, radiotherapy, and surgery compared with surgery alone for esophageal cancer: CALGB 9781. J Clin Oncol 2008;26(7):1086–92.

15. Iqbal S, McDonough S, Lenz HJ, et al. Randomized, phase ii study prospectively evaluating treatment of metastatic esophageal, gastric, or gastroesophageal cancer by gene expression of ERCC1: SWOG S1201. J Clin Oncol 2020;38(5):472–9.

16. Yang H, Liu H, Chen Y, et al. Long-term efficacy of neoadjuvant chemoradiotherapy plus surgery for the treatment of locally advanced esophageal squamous cell carcinoma: The NEOCRTEC5010 Randomized Clinical Trial. JAMA Surg 2021;156(8):721–9.

17. Reynolds JV, Preston SR, O'Neill B, et al. Neo-AEGIS (Neoadjuvant trial in Adenocarcinoma of the Esophagus and Esophago-Gastric Junction International Study): preliminary results of phase III RCT of CROSS versus perioperative chemotherapy (Modified MAGIC or FLOT protocol). (NCT01726452). J Clin Oncol 2021;39(15_suppl):4004.

18. Hoeppner J, Lordick F, Brunner T, et al. ESOPEC: prospective randomized controlled multicenter phase III trial comparing perioperative chemotherapy (FLOT protocol) to neoadjuvant chemoradiation (CROSS protocol) in patients with adenocarcinoma of the esophagus (NCT02509286). BMC Cancer 2016;16(1):503.

19. Stahl M, Stuschke M, Lehmann N, et al. Chemoradiation with and without surgery in patients with locally advanced squamous cell carcinoma of the esophagus. J Clin Oncol 2005;23(10):2310–7.

20. Bedenne L, Michel P, Bouché O, et al. Chemoradiation followed by surgery compared with chemoradiation alone in squamous cancer of the esophagus: FFCD 9102. J Clin Oncol 2007;25(10):1160–8.

21. Kelly RJ, Ajani JA, Kuzdzal J, et al. Adjuvant nivolumab in resected esophageal or gastroesophageal junction cancer. N Engl J Med 2021;384(13):1191–203.

22. Janjigian YY, Shitara K, Moehler M, et al. First-line nivolumab plus chemotherapy versus chemotherapy alone for advanced gastric, gastro-oesophageal junction, and oesophageal adenocarcinoma (CheckMate 649): a randomised, open-label, phase 3 trial. Lancet (London, England) 2021;398(10294):27–40.

23. Shah MA, Hofstetter WL, Kennedy EB, et al. Immunotherapy in patients with locally advanced esophageal carcinoma: ASCO treatment of locally advanced esophageal carcinoma guideline rapid recommendation update. J Clin Oncol 2021;39(28):3182–4.

24. Eggermont AMM, Blank CU, Mandala M, et al. Adjuvant pembrolizumab versus placebo in resected stage III melanoma. N Engl J Med 2018;378(19):1789–801.

25. Felip E, Altorki N, Zhou C, et al. Adjuvant atezolizumab after adjuvant chemotherapy in resected stage IB-IIIA non-small-cell lung cancer (IMpower010): a randomised, multicentre, open-label, phase 3 trial. Lancet 2021;398(10308):1344–57.

26. Bajorin DF, Witjes JA, Gschwend JE, et al. Adjuvant nivolumab versus placebo in muscle-invasive urothelial carcinoma. N Engl J Med 2021;384(22):2102–14.

27. Liu J, Blake SJ, Yong MC, et al. Improved efficacy of neoadjuvant compared to adjuvant immunotherapy to eradicate metastatic disease. Cancer Discov 2016;6(12):1382–99.

28. Boussiotis VA. Molecular and biochemical aspects of the PD-1 checkpoint pathway. N Engl J Med 2016;375(18):1767–78. Longo DL, ed.

29. Sato H, Niimi A, Yasuhara T, et al. DNA double-strand break repair pathway regulates PD-L1 expression in cancer cells. Nat Commun 2017;8(1):1751.

30. Li C, Zhao S, Zheng Y, et al. Preoperative pembrolizumab combined with chemoradiotherapy for oesophageal squamous cell carcinoma (PALACE-1). Eur J Cancer 2021;144:232–41.

31. Duan H, Shao C, Pan M, et al. Neoadjuvant pembrolizumab and chemotherapy in resectable esophageal cancer: an Open-Label, Single-Arm Study (PEN-ICE). Front Immunol 2022;13. 849984.

32. Shah MA, Bennouna J, Doi T, et al. KEYNOTE-975 study design: a Phase III study of definitive chemoradiotherapy plus pembrolizumab in patients with esophageal carcinoma. Future Oncol 2021;17(10): 1143–53.

33. Goodman KA, Xu R, Chau I, et al. SKYSCRAPER-07: A phase III, randomized, double-blind, placebo-controlled study of atezolizumab with or without tiragolumab in patients with unresectable ESCC who have not progressed following definitive concurrent chemoradiotherapy. J Clin Oncol 2022;40(4_suppl):TPS374.

34. Chauvin JM, Zarour HM. TIGIT in cancer immunotherapy. J Immunother Cancer 2020;8(2). e000957.

35. Cho BC, Abreu DR, Hussein M, et al. Tiragolumab plus atezolizumab versus placebo plus atezolizumab as a first-line treatment for PD-L1-selected non-small-cell lung cancer (CITYSCAPE): primary and follow-up analyses of a randomised, double-blind, phase 2 study. Lancet Oncol 2022;23(6):781–92.

36. Al-Batran S-E, Lorenzen S, Thuss-Patience PC, et al. Surgical and pathological outcome, and pathological regression, in patients receiving perioperative atezolizumab in combination with FLOT chemotherapy versus FLOT alone for resectable esophagogastric adenocarcinoma: Interim results from DANTE, a randomize. J Clin Oncol 2022;40(16_suppl):4003.

37. Janjigian YY, Van Cutsem E, Muro K, et al. MATTER-HORN: efficacy and safety of neoadjuvant-adjuvant durvalumab and FLOT chemotherapy in resectable gastric and gastroesophageal junction cancer—a randomized, double-blind, placebo-controlled, phase 3 study. J Clin Oncol 2021;39(15_suppl):TPS4151.

38. Eads JR, Weitz M, Gibson MK, et al. A phase II/III study of perioperative nivolumab and ipilimumab in patients (pts) with locoregional esophageal (E) and gastroesophageal junction (GEJ) adenocarcinoma: A trial of the ECOG-ACRIN Cancer Research Group (EA2174). J Clin Oncol 2020;38(15_suppl):TPS4651.

39. Terashima M, Kim Y-W, Yeh T-S, et al. ATTRACTION-05 (ONO-4538-38/BMS CA209844): a randomized, multicenter, double-blind, placebo- controlled Phase 3 study of Nivolumab (Nivo) in combination with adjuvant chemotherapy in pStage III gastric and esophagogastric junction (G/EGJ) cancer. Ann Oncol 2017;28:v266–7.

40. Bonneville R, Krook MA, Kautto EA, et al. Landscape of microsatellite instability across 39 cancer types. JCO Precis Oncol 2017;2017. https://doi.org/10.1200/PO.17.00073.

41. Vrána D, Matzenauer M, Neoral Č, et al. From tumor immunology to immunotherapy in gastric and esophageal cancer. Int J Mol Sci 2018;20(1):13.

42. Pietrantonio F, Miceli R, Raimondi A, et al. Individual patient data meta-analysis of the value of microsatellite instability as a biomarker in gastric cancer. J Clin Oncol 2019;37(35):3392–400.

43. André T, Tougeron D, Piessen G, et al. Neoadjuvant nivolumab plus ipilimumab and adjuvant nivolumab in localized deficient mismatch repair/microsatellite instability-high gastric or esophagogastric junction adenocarcinoma: The GERCOR NEONIPIGA Phase II Study. J Clin Oncol 2023;41(2):255–65.

44. Chatterton BE, Ho Shon I, Baldey A, et al. Positron emission tomography changes management and prognostic stratification in patients with oesophageal cancer: results of a multicentre prospective study. Eur J Nucl Med Mol Imaging 2009;36(3):354–61.

45. You JJ, Wong RKS, Darling G, et al. Clinical utility of 18F-Fluorodeoxyglucose positron emission tomography/computed tomography in the staging of patients with potentially resectable esophageal cancer. J Thorac Oncol 2013;8(12):1563–9.

46. Manabe O, Hattori N, Itoh K, et al. Value and limitation of 18F-FDG PET/CT in the staging of thoracic esophageal cancer. J Nucl Med 2011;52(1):1842.

47. Jiang C, Chen Y, Zhu Y, et al. Systematic review and meta-analysis of the accuracy of 18F-FDG PET/CT for detection of regional lymph node metastasis in esophageal squamous cell carcinoma. J Thorac Dis 2018;10(11):6066–76.

48. Cremonesi M, Garibaldi C, Timmerman R, et al. Interim 18 F-FDG-PET/CT during chemo-radiotherapy in the management of oesophageal cancer patients. A systematic review. Radiother Oncol 2017;125(2):200–12.

49. Weber WA, Ott K, Becker K, et al. Prediction of response to preoperative chemotherapy in adenocarcinomas of the esophagogastric junction by metabolic imaging. J Clin Oncol 2001;19(12):3058–65.

50. Ott K, Weber WA, Lordick F, et al. Metabolic imaging predicts response, survival, and recurrence in adenocarcinomas of the esophagogastric junction. J Clin Oncol 2006;24(29):4692–8.

51. Lordick F, Ott K, Krause B-J, et al. PET to assess early metabolic response and to guide treatment of adenocarcinoma of the oesophagogastric junction: the MUNICON phase II trial. Lancet Oncol 2007; 8(9):797–805.

52. Meyer zum Büschenfelde C, Herrmann K, Schuster T, et al. 18 F-FDG PET–guided salvage neoadjuvant radiochemotherapy of adenocarcinoma of the

esophagogastric junction: The MUNICON II Trial. J Nucl Med 2011;52(8):1189–96.

53. Barbour AP, Walpole ET, Mai GT, et al. Preoperative cisplatin, fluorouracil, and docetaxel with or without radiotherapy after poor early response to cisplatin and fluorouracil for resectable oesophageal adeno-carcinoma (AGITG DOCTOR): results from a multi-centre, randomised controlled phase II t. Ann Oncol 2020;31(2):236–45.

54. Lordick F, Herrmann K. Metabolic response assess-ment and PET-guided treatment of esophageal can-cer. Ann Oncol 2020;31(2):163–4.

55. Goodman KA, Ou F-S, Hall NC, et al. Randomized Phase II Study of PET response–adapted combined modality therapy for esophageal cancer: mature re-sults of the CALGB 80803 (Alliance) trial. J Clin On-col 2021;39(25):2803–15.

56. van Rossum PSN, Fried DV, Zhang L, et al. The value of 18F-FDG PET before and after induction chemotherapy for the early prediction of a poor pathologic response to subsequent preoperative chemoradiotherapy in oesophageal adenocarci-noma. Eur J Nucl Med Mol Imaging 2017;44(1):71–80.

57. Elimova E, Wang X, Etchebehere E, et al. 18-fluoro-deoxy-glucose positron emission computed tomogra-phy as predictive of response after chemoradiation in oesophageal cancer patients. Eur J Cancer 2015;51(17):2545–52.

58. Simoni N, Rossi G, Benetti G, et al. 18F-FDG PET/CT metrics are correlated to the pathological response in esophageal cancer patients treated with induction chemotherapy followed by neoadjuvant chemo-radiotherapy. Front Oncol 2020;10:1–11.

# Surgical Approach to Esophagectomy Post CheckMate 577
## Do Lymph Nodes Matter if Everyone Gets Adjuvant Immunotherapy?

Nikhil Panda, MD, MPH[a], Lana Schumacher, MD[b],*

**KEYWORDS**

• CheckMate 577 • Esophagectomy • Lymphadenectomy • Immunotherapy

**KEY POINTS**

• The standard of care for patients with locally advanced, resectable esophageal cancer is trimodality therapy with chemoradiotherapy followed by esophagectomy with lymphadenectomy.
• CheckMate 577 demonstrated a disease-free survival benefit among patients treated with adjuvant immunotherapy following trimodality therapy.
• In the era of adjuvant immunotherapy for patients with residual disease, the role of extended lymphadenectomy is unclear; potential improved locoregional control and appropriate pathologic staging continue to support lymphadenectomy at the time of esophagectomy.

## INTRODUCTION

The current standard of care for patients with locally advanced, resectable esophageal cancer is trimodality therapy with chemoradiotherapy followed by esophagectomy and lymphadenectomy. With this approach, 23% of patients with esophageal adenocarcinoma and 49% with esophageal squamous cell carcinoma experience a pathologic complete response, including patients with clinically node-positive, locally advanced disease.[1] Despite these results, patients remain at risk for disease recurrence. More than 30% of patients with residual disease following neoadjuvant chemoradiotherapy and esophagectomy experience local or, more frequently, distant recurrence.[2] As such, overall survival for patients with locally advanced, resectable esophageal cancer remains poor. In the 10-year outcome analysis of the original Chemoradiotherapy for Esophageal Cancer Followed by Surgery Study (CROSS) trial data, the 10-year overall survival among patients receiving trimodality therapy was 38%.[3] Taken together, there is a need for additional novel systemic therapy in the adjuvant setting, especially among patients without a pathologic complete response.

A growing body of literature has provided evidence for the use of immune checkpoint inhibitor therapy (I/O) in the treatment of advanced solid-organ malignancies, including esophageal cancer.[4,5] The addition of I/O may expand tumor-specific T-cells, enhance the cytotoxic effects of anti-tumor T-cells, and lead to biochemical changes within the tumor microenvironment to enhance the effects of chemotherapy and radiotherapy. CheckMate 577, a recent phase III randomized, double-blind, placebo-controlled trial

a Division of Thoracic Surgery, Department of Surgery, Massachusetts General Hospital, 55 Fruit Street, GRB-425, Boston, MA 02114, USA; b Division of Thoracic Surgery, Department of Surgery, Massachusetts General Hospital, 55 Fruit Street, Austen 7, Boston, MA, 02114, USA
* Corresponding author.
*E-mail address:* LSCHUMACHER2@mgh.harvard.edu
Twitter: @NikhilPanda_MD (N.P.)

Thorac Surg Clin 33 (2023) 209–213
https://doi.org/10.1016/j.thorsurg.2023.01.002

demonstrated a benefit in disease-free survival among patients with locally advanced, resectable esophageal cancer treated with adjuvant I/O following neoadjuvant chemoradiotherapy and esophagectomy.[6] CheckMate 577 marked the transition of I/O from the advanced to curative paradigm, and ongoing trials are further investigating the addition of I/O to neoadjuvant protocols.[7]

The results of the CheckMate 577 trial have been practice-changing in terms of clinical management. As a result, the debate around the need for and degree of extended lymphadenectomy at the time of esophagectomy has re-emerged. In terms of general oncologic principles, lymphadenectomy not only contributes toward locoregional control, but also accurate pathologic staging. However, the morbidity of extended lymphadenectomy, minimal pathologic upstaging, and questionable impact on clinical decision-making remain important considerations. In this review article, we discuss the surgical and oncologic considerations of extended lymphadenectomy at the time of esophagectomy for patients with locally advanced, resectable esophageal adenocarcinoma and squamous cell carcinoma. We then provide a review of CheckMate 577, the phase III trial demonstrating disease-free survival benefits of adjuvant I/O following neoadjuvant chemoradiotherapy and esophagectomy with lymphadenectomy. We conclude with a discussion of the pros and cons of extended lymphadenectomy at the time of esophagectomy, with acknowledgments to current and forthcoming innovations in thoracic surgery.

## BACKGROUND
### Anatomic Considerations

The lymphatic drainage of the esophagus has unique anatomic characteristics when considering tumor progression and metastases. There are rich networks of lymphatic channels that exist in nearly all layers of the esophagus (eg, lamina propria, muscularis mucosae, submucosa, circular and longitudinal muscle, and adventitia). In the inner layers (eg, lamina propria and submucosa), the lymphatic channels and drainage run primarily longitudinally along the length of the esophagus, but also radially through intermuscular channels.[8] As such, tumor cells can spread initially not only to locoregional lymph nodes (eg, peri-cardia gastric and posterior mediastinal lymph nodes), but also to distant paratracheal and cervical nodal basins. Tumors may spread to these distant lymph node basins in the absence of involved more proximal, locoregional lymph nodes, a phenomenon

known as "skipping.[9]" The presence of locoregional and distant lymph node metastases may occur early during the progression of mucosal lesions across the basement membrane of the epithelium. This is consistent with retrospective series of pathologic lymph node evaluation among patients with submucosal esophageal cancer, where the prevalence of lymph node metastases is approximately 20% among patients with adenocarcinoma and 35% among patients with squamous cell carcinoma.[10–12] The prevalence of lymph node metastases rapidly increases with further depth of invasion into the muscularis propria (30%–60%), adventitia (40%–80%), and adjacent structures (60%–100%).[13]

### Lymphadenectomy During Esophagectomy

Esophagectomy for esophageal cancer is accompanied by an extended lymphadenectomy for the oncologic purposes of locoregional control, accurate staging, and prognosis.[14] Differences in practice patterns and controversies remain in terms of the extent of lymphadenectomy, specifically two- versus three-field lymphadenectomy. The two-field lymphadenectomy includes the thorax (eg, paraesophageal, recurrent laryngeal nerves, subcarinal and hilar, diaphragmatic, and posterior mediastinal lymph nodes) and upper abdomen (eg, paracardial, lesser and greater curvature, left gastric, common hepatic, and celiac lymph nodes). A three-field lymphadenectomy includes these thoracic and upper abdominal lymph node basins, with the addition of cervical lymph nodes (eg, cervical paraesophageal and recurrent laryngeal nerves, deep cervical, and supraclavicular lymph nodes).[15] As expected, the three-field lymphadenectomy is associated with a higher lymph node yield, with conflicting data in terms of both the added morbidity of the cervical lymphadenectomy (eg, recurrent laryngeal nerve injury, chylothorax, pulmonary complications, and anastomotic leakage) and therapeutic value.[16,17]

Oncologic surgical principles suggest that resection of involved lymph nodes, assuming minimal morbidity, represents a form of locoregional control and contributes to improved disease-specific and overall survival. However, owing to the nature of early lymphatic spread and "skipping" lymph node stations for patients with esophageal cancer, these involved more distant lymph nodes (eg, deep cervical nodes) may represent a degree of systemic rather than locoregional metastases. In these cases, an extended two- or three-field lymphadenectomy may be of less benefit when considering potential additional operative morbidity. To explore this risk–benefit analysis, multiple observational studies have evaluated the optimal number of lymph nodes to resect at the time of an esophagectomy. In a systematic review and meta-analysis by Chen and colleagues of 12 studies evaluating the benefits of an extended lymphadenectomy among nearly 20,000 patients with esophageal adenocarcinoma and squamous cell carcinoma, a higher lymph node yield was associated with improved overall survival when up to 18 lymph nodes were resected.[17] The benefits were also observed in a subgroup analysis among patients who received neoadjuvant chemoradiotherapy. However, recent prospective, randomized data comparing two-versus three-field lymphadenectomy demonstrated no differences in the overall and disease-free survival.[9] In many of these studies, there are additional conflicting results in subgroup analyses when comparing histopathology (eg, squamous cell vs adenocarcinoma), the number of resected versus positive lymph nodes, and the receipt of neoadjuvant chemoradiotherapy.

With these data considered in western populations, the current recommendation by the National Comprehensive Cancer Network (NCCN) guidelines is that lymph node dissection should be performed in all patients regardless of receipt of neoadjuvant therapy for the purposes of identifying all potentially involved nodes and submitting at least 15 nodes for adequate pathologic staging.[18]

## CheckMate 577

The use of I/O in advanced (eg, unresectable or metastatic) esophageal squamous cell and adenocarcinoma is well described and is now a component of standard of care. ATTRACTION-3, a phase III trial comparing I/O versus chemotherapy among patients with previously treated advanced or recurrent esophageal cancer, demonstrated an improvement in overall survival among patients receiving I/O as second-line treatment following platinum- or fluoropyrimidine-based chemotherapy.[4] CheckMate 648 was a recent phase III trial evaluating the use of combined chemotherapy and I/O as first-line treatment of patients with previously untreated, unresectable esophageal cancer and demonstrated an overall survival benefit compared with chemotherapy alone.[5]

CheckMate 577 was a randomized, double-blind, placebo-controlled phase III trial evaluating the use of I/O as adjuvant treatment among patients with esophageal or gastroesophageal junction cancer who underwent neoadjuvant chemoradiotherapy followed by esophagectomy.[6] The I/O intervention was Nivolumab, a human

monoclonal anti-programmed death-1 (PD-1) antibody. PD-1 is a T-cell receptor that, when bound to programmed death ligand-1 (PDL-1) on tumor cells, functions as a negative regulator of cytotoxic, anti-tumor effects. As such, Nivolumab binds to the PD-1 receptor, preventing the PD-1/PDL-1 interaction and promotes the anti-tumor effects of host T-cells.

A notable component of the study design was a prespecified stratified randomization by positive pathologic lymph nodes. The surgical approaches and extent of lymphadenectomy data for the included patients were not provided from the sites across the 29 countries that participated in the trial. The primary endpoint was disease-free survival. Among the 794 patients who underwent randomization, 262 received placebo and 532 received Nivolumab. The primary histologic subtype was adenocarcinoma (71% in both cohorts) and most patients had pathologic nodal involvement ($\geq$ypN1 57% in Nivolumab and 58% in placebo cohorts). The disease-free survival was longer among patients who received Nivolumab compared with placebo (22.4 vs 11.0 months, unstratified hazard ratio [HR] 0.69). Interestingly, in the prespecified subgroup analysis comparing disease-free survival of patients with and without positive lymph nodes, Nivolumab was favored only among patients with positive lymph nodes (unstratified HR 0.67).

## DISCUSSION POINTS

In May 2021, the use of adjuvant Nivolumab was approved by the Food and Drug Administration and remains an NCCN category level one recommendation for patients without a pathologic complete response following neoadjuvant chemoradiotherapy and esophagectomy. In short, patients with ypT + or ypN + disease should be considered for adjuvant I/O therapy. Given the promising results of CheckMate 577, the debate around the need for and extent of lymphadenectomy at the time of esophagectomy has re-emerged: does the lymph node yield matter if most patients will receive adjuvant I/O? Salient discussion points are organized below.

### The "Pros"

Arguments for performing an extended lymphadenectomy at the time of esophagectomy in the adjuvant I/O era continue to include the fundamental oncologic principle of improved locoregional control. The CheckMate 577 data did not allow a further subgroup analysis among the 457 $\geq$ypN1 patients to specifically evaluate the benefits of adjuvant I/O by extent of lymphadenectomy. As such, disease-free and overall survival data demonstrating non-inferiority of adjuvant I/O following a limited lymphadenectomy remain lacking. In addition, an extended lymphadenectomy allows for appropriate pathologic staging. Many may argue that this consideration is irrelevant given patients with ypT+ and ypN + disease are candidates for adjuvant I/O. However, an adequate lymphadenectomy will identify patients with a pathologic complete response who require no additional adjuvant therapy. In addition, appropriate pathologic staging has an impact on prognostication in terms of benefits of adjuvant I/O (eg, CheckMate 577 patients with $\geq$ypN1 disease experienced a survival benefit with adjuvant I/O), as well as survival.

### The "Cons"

In contrast to the benefits outlined above, the key argument against performing an extended lymphadenectomy at the time of esophagectomy is the limited impact on clinical decision-making. Following CheckMate 577 and the Food and Drug Administration approval of adjuvant Nivolumab, the NCCN guidelines recommend that all patients with ypT + or ypN + disease be considered for adjuvant I/O. Although there are patients who will experience a complete pathologic response, most patients have a residual disease or remain at risk for recurrence. A second consideration is that despite the innovations made in novel systemic therapy for esophageal cancer, pathobiology and patterns of tumor metastasis continue to remain unclear. Taken together, the morbidity of additional lymph node harvest at the time of esophagectomy may outweigh the clinical and oncologic benefits.

### Future Considerations

In summary, the role of an extended lymphadenectomy at the time of esophagectomy following neoadjuvant chemoradiotherapy for patients with locally advanced esophageal cancer remains unknown. There are several exciting areas of ongoing research that are likely to allow clinicians to revisit the benefits of extended lymphadenectomy at the time of esophagectomy in the I/O era. There is an existing and growing body of data evaluating the role of various surgical approaches, especially robotic-assisted esophagectomy, on the yield and morbidity of an extended lymphadenectomy. There are conflicting results, where some data support a higher lymph node yield following robotic-assisted surgery and other show no difference and comparable surgical morbidity.[19] The individual studies are limited by small sample sizes

and observational study designs, and there are likely surgeon, patient, and disease-specific considerations behind these conflicting results. However, robotic platforms do allow for a seamless implementation of emerging navigational and localization technology. These innovations may improve not only the yield of lymph nodes, but also the identification of the appropriate lymph node basins for inclusion in extended lymphadenectomy.[20–22] In addition to surgical innovation, I/O regimens are now being integrated into neoadjuvant protocols alongside chemoradiotherapy.[23] Preliminary data suggest no additional morbidity of extended lymphadenectomy in I/O-treated lymph node basins. An extended lymphadenectomy will remain critical to understanding the efficacy of neoadjuvant I/O, contributions to locoregional control, and decision-making for adjuvant therapy.

For these reasons, we recommend an extended (ie, at least 15 lymph nodes) lymphadenectomy at the time of esophagectomy for esophageal cancer for improved locoregional control and appropriate pathologic staging. Among experienced thoracic surgeons, we feel these clinical and oncologic benefits are provided with minimal additional morbidity to patients. Furthermore, current and forthcoming surgical and oncologic innovations—namely robotic and localization technologies as well as neoadjuvant I/O regimens—will further allow clinicians to understand the role and therapeutic value of an extended lymphadenectomy at the time of esophagectomy.

## DISCLOSURES

The authors have nothing to disclose.

## REFERENCES

1. van Hagen P, Hulshof MCCM, van Lanschot JJB, et al. Preoperative Chemoradiotherapy for Esophageal or Junctional Cancer. N Engl J Med 2012; 366(22):2074–84.
2. Blum Murphy M, Xiao L, Patel VR, et al. Pathological complete response in patients with esophageal cancer after the trimodality approach: The association with baseline variables and survival—The University of Texas MD Anderson Cancer Center experience. Cancer 2017;123(21):4106–13.
3. Eyck BM, van Lanschot JJB, Hulshof MCCM, et al. Ten-Year Outcome of Neoadjuvant Chemoradiotherapy Plus Surgery for Esophageal Cancer: The Randomized Controlled CROSS Trial. J Clin Oncol 2021; 39(18):1995–2004.
4. Kato K, Cho BC, Takahashi M, et al. Nivolumab versus chemotherapy in patients with advanced

oesophageal squamous cell carcinoma refractory or intolerant to previous chemotherapy (ATTRACTION-3): a multicentre, randomised, open-label, phase 3 trial. Lancet Oncol 2019;20(11):1506–17.

5. Doki Y, Ajani JA, Kato K, et al. Nivolumab Combination Therapy in Advanced Esophageal Squamous-Cell Carcinoma. N Engl J Med 2022;386(5):449–62.

6. Kelly RJ, Ajani JA, Kuzdzal J, et al. Adjuvant Nivolumab in Resected Esophageal or Gastroesophageal Junction Cancer. N Engl J Med 2021;384(13): 1191–203.

7. Sihag S, Ku GY, Tan KS, et al. Safety and feasibility of esophagectomy following combined immunotherapy and chemoradiotherapy for esophageal cancer. J Thorac Cardiovasc Surg 2021;161(3): 836–43.e1.

8. Wang Y, Zhu L, Xia W, et al. Anatomy of lymphatic drainage of the esophagus and lymph node metastasis of thoracic esophageal cancer. Cancer Manag Res 2018;10:6295.

9. Li B, Zhang Y, Miao L, et al. Esophagectomy With Three-Field Versus Two-Field Lymphadenectomy for Middle and Lower Thoracic Esophageal Cancer: Long-Term Outcomes of a Randomized Clinical Trial. J Thorac Oncol 2021;16(2):310–7.

10. Stein HJ, Feith M, Bruecher BLDM, et al. Early Esophageal Cancer: Pattern of Lymphatic Spread and Prognostic Factors for Long-Term Survival After Surgical Resection. Ann Surg 2005;242(4):566.

11. Buskens CJ, Westerterp M, Lagarde SM, et al. Prediction of appropriateness of local endoscopic treatment for high-grade dysplasia and early adenocarcinoma by EUS and histopathologic features. Gastrointest Endosc 2004;60(5):703–10.

12. Rice TW, Blackstone EH, Goldblum JR, et al. Superficial adenocarcinoma of the esophagus. J Thorac Cardiovasc Surg 2001;122(6):1077–90.

13. Cho JW, Choi SC, Jang JY, et al. Lymph Node Metastases in Esophageal Carcinoma: An Endoscopist's View. Clin Endosc 2014;47(6):523.

14. Kingma BF, Ruurda JP, van Hillegersberg R. An Editorial on Lymphadenectomy in Esophagectomy for Cancer. Ann Surg Oncol 2022;29(8):4676–8.

15. Nafteux P, Depypere L, Veer H Van, et al. Principles of esophageal cancer surgery, including surgical approaches and optimal node dissection (2- vs . 3-field). Ann Cardiothorac Surg 2017;6(2):15258.

16. Tachibana M, Kinugasa S, Yoshimura H, et al. Extended Esophagectomy With 3-Field Lymph Node Dissection for Esophageal Cancer. Arch Surg 2003;138(12):1383–9.

17. Chen D, Mao Y, Xue Y, et al. Does the lymph node yield affect survival in patients with esophageal cancer receiving neoadjuvant therapy plus esophagectomy? A systematic review and updated meta-analysis. EClinicalMedicine 2020;25:100431.

18. McMillian N, Lenora Pluchino MA, Ajani JA, et al. NCCN Guidelines Version 4.2022 Esophageal and Esophagogastric Junction Cancers. 2022. Available at: https://www.nccn.org/home/. Accessed September 13, 2022.

19. Domene CE, Volpe P. Do robotic arms retrieve more lymph nodes during an esophagectomy? Ann Esophagus 2020;3(0). https://doi.org/10.21037/AOE.2020.02.03.

20. Wang X, Hu Y, Wu X, et al. Near-infrared fluorescence imaging-guided lymphatic mapping in thoracic esophageal cancer surgery. Surg Endosc 2022;36(6):3994–4003.

21. Hachey KJ, Gilmore DM, Armstrong KW, et al. Safety and feasibility of near-infrared image-guided lymphatic mapping of regional lymph nodes in esophageal cancer. J Thorac Cardiovasc Surg 2016;152(2):546–54.

22. Jimenez-Lillo J, Villegas-Tovar E, Momblan-Garcia D, et al. Performance of Indocyanine-Green Imaging for Sentinel Lymph Node Mapping and Lymph Node Metastasis in Esophageal Cancer: Systematic Review and Meta-Analysis. Ann Surg Oncol 2021;28(9):4869–77.

23. Sihag S, Kosinski AS, Gaissert HA, et al. Minimally Invasive Versus Open Esophagectomy for Esophageal Cancer: A Comparison of Early Surgical Outcomes from the Society of Thoracic Surgeons National Database. Ann Thorac Surg 2016;101(4): 1281–9.

# Moving?

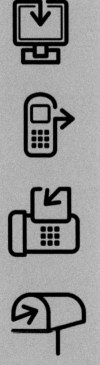